The ULTIMATE GUIDE to SEDUCTION & FOREPLAY

The ULTIMATE GUIDE to SEDUCTION & FOREPLAY

TECHNIQUES AND STRATEGIES FOR MIND-BLOWING SEX

JESSICA O'REILLY, PhD &
MARLA RENEE STEWART, MA

Published in the United States by Cleis Press, an imprint of Start Midnight, LLC, 221 River Street, Ninth Floor, Hoboken NJ 07030.

Printed in the United States
Cover design: Allyson Fields
Cover image: iStock
Text design: Frank Wiedemann
First Edition
10 9 8 7 6 5 4 3 2 1

Trade paper ISBN: 978-1-62778-298-2
E-book ISBN: 978-1-62778-511-2

CONTENTS

WHAT IS FOREPLAY?
WHAT IS SEDUCTION?

When presented with the opportunity to write this book, we had a thoughtful conversation about how we define seduction, foreplay, and sex. Mainstream (read: heteronormative) audiences tend to believe that foreplay involves everything you do before you engage in penis-in-vagina sex, which might include kissing, touching, hand stimulation of the genitals, and even oral sex. However, when you engage in manual sex or oral sex, you refer to both activities as *sex*, so it follows that seduction and foreplay *are* types of sex. They are also part of the escalation to what (you hope) will be a fulfilling sexual experience.

The fact is that sex means different things to different people, and it is up to you to determine what sex means to you. If you believe that sex is comprised of all erotic encounters, including the seduction of the mind, you are right. If you define sex as the act of putting the penis in the vagina, you are also right. And if you define sex as the euphoric feeling of pleasure and intimacy you cultivate when you connect emotionally and physically with your lover(s), you too are correct. What is more important is how you approach sex with your lover(s) to ensure that you are on the same sexual wavelength.

You don't have to be a rock star in the bedroom each and every time you have sex, but we can all benefit from approaching our lovers with confidence before, during, and after sex—however you define it.

Seduction and foreplay may be one and the same. They may overlap, and they may blend into a seamless experience of sexual delight. Because of pickup culture, some folks may have come to associate seduction with manipulative tactics aimed at pressuring or swindling someone into hooking up or having sex; pickup artists use the language of seduction but conflate it with control, deception, and dishonesty. This is not our version of seduction and we know that it is not yours either. When we talk about seduction, we put consent and mutual desire at its core. Seduction is not about getting what you want; seduction involves both giving and receiving pleasure of all kinds so that all parties involved reap the ultimate sexual (and nonsexual) rewards.

In the upcoming chapters, we share seduction and foreplay approaches, techniques, and methods ranging from verbal and emotional seduction to physical touch and oral sex. We also address practical strategies related to confidence and daily interactions—all of which are intended to make seduction and foreplay more exciting and approachable. But **you do not have to do it all.** The key for you, as the reader, involves identifying the strategies and approaches that align with your needs and your lovers'. Your personalities, desires, and values will all influence how you respond to these potential tools, and your needs will evolve over time.

No two lovers are identical, so there are no surefire approaches or tips that will universally make any lover quiver with desire and pleasure. This means that you do not have to master everything at once, nor do you need to embrace every tip and technique.

You are the ultimate expert in your own sex life, so if something doesn't work for you, don't force it. Your sexual options are endless, and if you keep an open mind, embrace feedback, and experiment with new sexual experiences, you will discover thrilling pathways to pleasure and intimacy.

Throughout the text, we have included a series of action items for you to try on your own or with your partner(s). Take your time to work through the exercises and activities. There's no rush, as these suggestions can be used today, adapted tomorrow, and refined in the upcoming weeks, months, and years.

If you are currently in a relationship, you might use these action items as part of your daily or weekly check-ins, and regardless of relationship status, consider setting reminders in your calendar to return to these activities again in two to three months. Weaving some of these items into your daily or weekly routines will help you to prioritize your relationship(s) and make intimacy and eroticism a part of your regular interactions.

Seduction Instructions are homework assignments that you can do on your own or with your lover(s). They include personal journals and reflections, partnered activities, and physical touch exercises. We encourage you to repeat these assignments more than once to continue learning about yourself and your lover(s).

Tantalizing Tips include extra information or variations to make your experiences hotter, sexier, and more inventive.

Lovers' Inquiries are questionnaires and interviews that you complete with your partner(s). They are intended to improve understanding and deepen connection to enhance your sexual and seductive prowess.

We hope that you will put theory into practice starting today and follow through for years to come. If you are here, we know you are already ahead of the game and you have embraced the growth mindset, so without further ado, let us dive in and get started.

SEDUCTION INSTRUCTION

Start thinking about your understandings of sex, seduction, and foreplay by answering the following questions or using them as prompts to write in your journal. If you prefer not to write, you can use the voice-to-text function or voice notes app on your phone to record your thoughts. If you use voice-to-text, you can reread your response and make edits and additions as you review the text.

- How do you define sex?
- How do you think your lover(s) define(s) sex? Is this a conversation you have addressed or want to address in the future?
- How do you define seduction and foreplay?
- How do you think your lover(s) define(s) seduction and foreplay?
- What would you like to learn about seduction and foreplay?
- What do you find challenging about seduction and foreplay?

Seduction at a Glance

Seduction can be the most alluring and the most challenging part of sex. Once we get started, sex can flow freely and naturally, but seducing a lover and initiating sex can sometimes feel intimidating and awkward. The transition from your daily routine to a sexual interaction may feel unsophisticated, and your subconscious fear of rejection can deter you from making a move. Some folks overthink seduction and are faced with paralysis by analysis, and others struggle to gauge their lovers' interest in sex, leaving them unsure as to whether or not the timing is right. The good news is that each of these challenges is surmountable.

Seduction refers to the art of teasing and pleasing, but it is also about enticing others to be curious about you while simultaneously catering to their desires. Seduction involves making a gracious offer to pique their interest free from pressure. The mind plays an important role in seduction, and seduction exists in all types of relationships.

A master seducer not only seduces people that they want to sleep with, but they also have the natural ability to charm friends, coworkers, their children, and other family members because they realize that seduction is not always about eroticism—it is a state of mind. It involves influencing people in a way that benefits all parties—a negotiation of sorts without the formalities. It is a way of invoking the best traits of your personality and catering to your audience in a manner that taps in to their most intimate desires. And, of course, the power of seduction is always underscored by consent and should be free from coercion regardless of the type of relationship.

Those who have mastered the art and skill of seduction tend to share a number of important traits, attitudes, and approaches. We've summarized these as the **seven statutes of seduction** that underpin and inform the strategies outlined in the upcoming chapters.

The Seven Statutes of Seduction

Build anticipation. Anticipation is not the precursor to pleasure; *anticipation is pleasure.* If you go straight for the goods (e.g., reach down their pants right away), you will both miss out on this important stage of pleasure; whereas if you take the time to allude to all the ways you want to touch them with your words, body language, and teasing touch, you build sexual energy and desire that mounts into a more climactic response.

Research suggests that dopamine, a chemical associated with reward, pleasure, and motivation, is released as soon as we begin to anticipate a reward—not just when we receive it. This is why planning a vacation is often more exciting and pleasurable than the trip itself and why dopamine levels can rise dramatically when we dream of future plans like retirement.

Robert Sapolsky's study of monkeys found that dopamine spikes as soon as the possibility of a reward arises and the release ends when the reward is received, suggesting that the *pursuit* of pleasure results in the chemical release. Sapolsky trained monkeys to respond to a light by pressing a lever and receiving a (food) reward. Over time, the monkeys experienced the dopamine spike in response to the light alone, as the anticipation was enough to induce the chemical response. What's more, when they changed things up so that the reward was only received 50 percent of the time, dopamine levels increased even more significantly.[1] The takeaway is that excitement of the unknown produces a more significant response than the guarantee of the reward itself.

It follows that the most memorable and exciting seduction involves cultivating desire over time and employing multiple approaches to remain unpredictable. This is why you do not master seduction by learning a specific technique, but by being open to multiple approaches, including those that may fall outside your comfort zone.

Show curiosity. Seduction involves piquing the curiosity of your lover(s), and one of the best ways to do this is to let them know that you want to know more about them. Ask them what they want. Really listen as though it's the first time you are learning about sexual seduction and pleasure—especially if you feel you already know them. Prioritize their feedback over anything you can learn from a book or previous lovers.

Just as the most likable people are those who show interest in others by asking them about their lives and experiences, the most desired lovers derive pleasure from learning about others for the sake of discovery—not performance. When you ask your lover for guidance and feedback, embrace the process of learning and gaining insights into their sexual fingerprint as opposed to trying to convert the information into a specific technique you can use right away. When you make the love of learning a part of your sex play, the pleasure and discovery can last a lifetime.

Let less be more. You do not need to *do the most* when it comes to seduction. Seduction is a slow process that you can curate to suit your own needs, so take your time and allow your words, touch, and actions to flow freely. You can always use new strategies and techniques, but don't get hung up on implementing them perfectly or utilizing them all at once. A gentle brush of the thigh in the morning can go just as far as creating a complex erotic lair that requires thirty minutes of setup. Do what works for you. You do not want sex to become a chore or another item you have to check off your task list.

Be present and mindful. You are more attractive when you are in the moment and focused on the interaction at hand. When you are mindful of your lover(s), the environment, your own body, and all of the associated sensations, pleasure skyrockets. Presence simply refers to being in the moment—not in the past and not in the future, but right here, right now. When you are present, you are not worried about what is happening in the next room, you are not concerned about how you look, you are not concerned about your technique, you are not wondering what other people are thinking. When you are present, you show up for your partner(s), and they feel valued, prioritized, and desired.

Being mindful involves being present in the moment without judgment. You might be comfortable or uncomfortable at any given moment, but that doesn't make it good or bad. It just is. We spend a good degree of our lives moving through the world mindlessly, but we do not want mindless relationships or mindless sex. Mindful connections and mindful sex are associated with heightened desire, lower performance anxiety, and enhanced sexual response—all of which create the potential for more intense pleasure.

Be on the lookout for specific mindfulness exercises in the chapter "Mindful Touch and Seduction for Busy People."

Do not take everything personally. Sometimes, it's not about you. Be humble and gracious in your understanding of your lover(s) and accept that if they do not respond to your advances, it may have nothing to do with you. They are not required to offer an explanation that satisfies your needs. If you take things personally, you are less likely to put yourself out there and may avoid initiating seduction altogether. Be aware of your own thoughts and feelings and accept that you can only adjust your own behavior—not your partner's.

The best lovers communicate their desires, feelings, and boundaries. But this does not mean that you are entitled to know everything about your partner. Some mystery will always remain, and this can be both frustrating and exciting—tap in to the latter instead of focusing on the former, and you will be a better seducer, lover, and partner.

Embrace rejection so that you expand your comfort zone and take risks. Let's face it: we are all afraid of being rejected, but those who look at the possibility of rejection as a challenge rather than a deterrent make the best lovers. Rejection is part of life, love, and sex, and it can be painful. Your brain's response to social pain like rejection is similar to its response to physical pain. This physical brain response is so strong that one study found that taking acetaminophen prior to recalling an emotionally painful experience can reduce the emotional pain.* Rejection can wreak havoc on your mood, health habits, self-esteem, and even cognitive functioning.

However, learning to manage rejection makes for more fulfilling relationships than trying to avoid rejection altogether. If you only do things that you are immediately comfortable with, you are less likely to grow and experience fulfillment. Whereas if you learn to manage rejection, you are more likely to take risks and expand your comfort zone. You will learn from past experiences (including sexual rejection) and adjust your approach and behavior moving forward.

For example, you might try to flirt with your lover while they are making dinner and find that they shut you down when you kiss them on the neck; from this you might learn that your flirtation needs to begin earlier in the day to cultivate connection, or that helping with dinner will lower their stress and make them more open to your advances. Or they might communicate to you that they do not like to be kissed on the neck when they're cooking because they're sweaty, but they like being caressed through their clothing.

This is a very simple example, but the possibilities are endless when it comes to learning from rejection, and you might find that you begin to reframe the idea of rejection into a learning opportunity as opposed to a letdown. Your partner didn't say no to sex—

---

* We are not suggesting that you take medicine to address painful feelings, but simply noting the ways in which the effects of emotional pain can mirror those associated with physical pain.

they showed you how to make sex more likely and pleasurable.

If you avoid rejection, you will inevitably hold back and miss out on opportunities—in life and in sexual relationships. If you embrace it as an opportunity for challenge and revelation, you will not only have more sex, but you will discover so many new things about yourself, your lover(s), and sexual pleasure.

Keep an open mind. You do not have to be into everything, but don't assume that your norm is *the* norm. Just because a sex act or experience is unappealing to you doesn't mean someone else (including your partner) cannot derive extreme pleasure from it. There are no universal rules when it comes to sex and relationships, so be open to considering options beyond what immediately appeals to you. If you reject an idea from the onset, you will miss out on all of the related intricacies and details that might be immensely pleasurable for both you and your partner(s).

For example, perhaps your lover is interested in attending a sex club—not to participate, but just to watch. The idea makes you uncomfortable. You have no interest in going. You can reply with judgment: *That's gross. It's perverted. All the people will be unattractive.* Or you can reply with an open mind: *The thought of a sex club makes me really uncomfortable, but I'm open to learning more. What makes you want to go? What have you heard about them? What's the appeal for you? What might the appeal be for me? Is there a place I can read to learn a bit more and have some questions answered? I'm not comfortable going at this time, but I'd like to keep talking about it.*

Having an open mind doesn't mean that you have to do more when it comes to sex, but being willing to learn, considering alternative perspectives, and talking about a range of experiences (including those beyond your comfort zone) will make you a better partner and seducer as you learn to weave elements of your lover's desires into your seduction routine.

While some folks cannot help but ooze seduction in every inter-action, others struggle with habits and attitudes that are inher-ently anti-seductive.

For example, being self-absorbed is generally a turnoff. Social media hype means that taking and posting photos of ourselves, bragging about experiences, and comparing ourselves to others' highlight reels is the norm. And while there are benefits to loving yourself, celebrating your achievements, and showing off a little, too much can be a turnoff. Offline, if you always talk about yourself at the expense of paying attention to others, it can be difficult for your lover(s) to recognize and respond to your seductive advances. We all believe that we are here to share our gifts with the world and have the world share their gifts with us, but if you believe or act as though you know it all, you are bound to overpromise and underdeliver.

Similarly, if you make moral judgments about other people, it can be antiseductive. You are entitled to your opinions and pref-erences, but if you refuse to open your mind to others, it will cost you in relationships of all types. If you waste your energy talking about and judging what other people do, whom they sleep with, what they wear, or how they live their lives, it is generally unsexy and antiseductive. Just because something doesn't appeal to you doesn't mean that it will not appeal to others. It's natural to assess the appeal of a sexual scenario or partner (e.g., I do or do not find that attractive), but when you yuck someone else's yum, your own appeal plummets.

Likewise, if you play games or shut down ideas that make you uncomfortable, this can also quash desire and seduction. If something doesn't immediately appeal to you, that is okay and you have a right to express your dislike or discomfort. You can also clearly delineate your boundaries to your lover(s). But it is equally important to validate your lovers' interests even if they differ from your own. For example, perhaps they playfully propose going skinny dipping and express that running around naked in the dark helps to set the mood for eroticism, but you are just not into it. Do you respond with judgment to shut them down? *Stop it. You are so immature. I'm not going!* Or do you respond graciously and honestly? *I'm not into cold-water naked swims. But can I come cheer you on from the dock or meet you in the shower when you are done?* Part of being adept at seduction also involves learning to be seduced, so the way you respond to their flirtatious, playful, and seductive advances is as important as how you initiate.

Seduction is multifaceted, dynamic, and highly personal, so you can slip up with antiseductive behavior at times and, of course, make up for it later. Go easy on yourself and enjoy being authentic, thoughtful, playful, mysterious, open-minded—and imperfect.

SEDUCTION INSTRUCTION

Answer the following questions or use them as free-writing prompts in your journal:

▶ What is the most seductive thing about you?

▶ What have other people told you about your sex appeal? What do they say turns them on when it comes to your personality, behavior, or appearance?

▶ What behaviors make you antiseductive? Would you like to change anything about your behavior or approach?

▶ What do people find curious about you? How do you entice others to be curious about you?

▸ Do you consider yourself open-minded? Is there anything you would like to work on when it comes to keeping an open mind?

▸ How do you handle rejection? How did you respond the last time you faced rejection (not limited to sex)? Do you want to adjust the way you think or behave moving forward?

▸ Do you tend to take things personally? What might you do differently in the future?

▸ Do you find that you are present and mindful when you spend time with your lover(s) or on your own? What helps you to stay in the moment? What detracts you from being mindful and present?

A Brief but Important Note About Safer Sex

Many of the techniques and approaches we cover suggest skin-to-skin contact and may involve being with a partner with whom you are fluid bonded. Any time you engage in any type of sex, we recommend that you practice safer sex. This includes, but is not limited to, the use of contraception, barriers, and harm-reduction techniques to reduce the risk of sexually transmitted infections and other outcomes you wish to limit or avoid.

Barrier method options include external condoms, internal condoms, gloves, and dental dams. If you have long nails, put cotton balls in the fingertips of gloves to reduce the likelihood of tearing. You can also use gloves to create your own dental dams: cut the fingers off and leave the thumb intact. Cut all the way up the side opposite the thumb to open it up, and use the thumb for insertions or slide your tongue inside.

Safer sex, of course, also requires communication and a consideration of emotional safety. Talk about your testing routines and consider getting tested together. Be honest about your desires and intentions. Prior to engaging in sexual activity, consider a range of scenarios and interactions that might occur and think (and talk) about how you might respond emotionally.

This is not an exhaustive list. We encourage you to practice safer sex according to your specific needs in order to reduce harm and risk for all parties involved. Check out Scarleteen's website for some incredible insights about safer sex in all sorts of different scenarios: https://www.scarleteen.com/tags/safer_sex.

SEDUCTION FANTASIES

When it comes to foreplay, seduction, and sex, you can learn from experience, learn from your partner, and learn from the so-called experts like us. But we believe that the most valuable learning occurs when you get a glimpse into a range of real experiences and preferences—even if they are not all to your liking. So we asked our communities to share their ultimate seduction fantasies, because we cannot do this on our own. When it comes to sex, none of us is a universal expert. As sex researchers, it's our job to study, listen, and learn on a daily basis, but our expertise will always fall short in comparison to *your own* experience. You are the ultimate expert in your own pleasure.

This is why we love hearing and learning from you. Your stories are varied and vivid, and we can all draw inspiration from one another in so many ways. Of course, one person's fantasy is another's nightmare, so as you read through these submissions, keep an open mind and consider which elements appeal to you and which ones are not currently your cup of tea.

As always, remember not to yuck someone else's yum. Just because you do not fancy a particular approach doesn't mean it lacks value or substance. And more importantly, what appeals to you may be different from what appeals to your partner(s), so explore and draw from an array of approaches and fantasies to help you to better understand and meet one another's needs.

As we say in the kink community, your kink isn't my kink, but your kink is okay.

As you read through your friends' and neighbors' fantasies below, pay attention to your own reactions—emotional, physical, visceral, and erotic. There is no right way to respond, and you may be surprised by what turns you on and turns you off, so allow your reactions to arise without inhibition or self-censure.

Real Fantasies from
Your Friends and Neighbors

She makes me laugh all night long. We laugh hard over dinner, over drinks, and then on the car ride home. When we get into bed, she's still joking around. The whole thing is playful. We do not stop laughing. Without totally undressing me, she licks my whole body—almost like a cat. It is not serious like in the movies. It is not sexy in the sense of porn, but it is sexy because we giggle so much. The fun makes it intense. At some point, she turns on my vibrator but leaves it on the bedside table so I can hear it. It is not coming yet. The whole time, she is laughing, and it makes me laugh too. I've always been nervous about sex. It was so taboo in my house growing up, so even though I know I should relax, I still haven't overcome all of my hang-ups. Laughing makes the tension and nerves subside. We are kissing and giggling and almost rolling around laughing before we really get down to it. Hilarity is seduction at its finest, in my opinion.

B.H., 40

She doesn't talk at all. I just walk in the door, and she can see that I've had a hard day. She turns the TV on for the kids and walks upstairs. I follow, and she's waiting in the shower. I walk in, and she gets out all wet and starts undressing me. She isn't hiding her body or worrying about the lights like she usually does. She has it all on display without a hint of self-consciousness. She has never been so hot. My suit gets wet, and she just keeps going, dropping to her knees to suck me hard just for a minute. She sits up on the sink and grabs my hair, forcing me down between her legs. I lick around for a short while and then slide inside her without a word. We're quiet and quick and we never talk about it, even though we know it will happen again.

Toni, 39

I just want to be woken up with a blow job. It doesn't matter who does it. Gender doesn't matter. I just want that morning surprise.

Kris, 24

Seduction is without a doubt the hottest part of sex for me. Sex always feels good, but the buildup is what really makes the difference for me. I want him to eat me alive with his eyes and not be shy about it or make me feel shy in return. Really *look* at me like he wants to devour me all through dinner. I want him to tell me that he cannot wait to get out of the restaurant because he *needs* me. I just bite my lip and smile a little, but he keeps asking when we can leave. If he really shows his *desperation* for me, I'm easily seduced.

Kiki, 31

I just want to be touched. We often talk about taking your time with a woman's body to really explore it, but as a guy, I want the same thing. I want her to come on to me and touch me all over. I don't care about the technique as long as she takes the initiative.

Adrian, 40

I love to be teased and touched all over. I want to beg for it; I want to need it. I want to be dominated either kindly and softly or more aggressively depending on my mood and the situation—but I always like a little bit of domination and pain (biting, spanking, grabbing). I want it to start off sweet and passionate, light and soft, and depending on the situation, either slowly becoming more aggressive with teasing, or just completely dominating me. I want my legs to be caressed and for them to slowly move up my body. I want it to be soft but with a touch of aggression—tickle my legs and inner thigh, but grab and spank my ass. Kiss me all over, from my lips to my neck to my nipples (spend some time there) and play with my breasts for a bit. Then kiss and caress your way down to my lower abdomen, teasing me by kissing and licking all around my vulva, but not giving me head yet. I love finger play (sometimes more than intercourse) so I'd want them to slowly finger me, then perform oral sex. Then stop oral and just finger me while watching me be turned on—then have sex.

Anna, 23

I just want deep conversations. I want a partner who really listens and is willing to get deep into the real conversations—not small talk, but the serious, intense topics like politics and human philosophy. It's a brain-first thing for me when it comes to sex.

Aja, 32

It is funny how your love language translates into the bedroom. I like acts of service, and they are also my ultimate turn-on. I'd love to walk in the door and have her greet me and lead me to a chair. She would drop to her knees and help take off my boots. If she were to bring me a drink or hang up my coat, it would take it to the next level. I'm not expecting her to do any of these things because she's a woman or anything like that. I just find that when she does stuff like this (and it is out of the ordinary), I get so turned on.

Les, 36

I like when he strokes himself while he's waiting for me to come to bed. There's nothing hotter than seeing him hard and standing at attention when I walk in. I slip off my robe, and he moans and touches himself some more while he looks me over. . .

Olga, 29

I want to be a good girl, so if my lover plays with that during the day, I'll be aching for it and willing to do whatever when I get home after work. I like when she sends me texts telling me how good I was last night or earlier in the week. Basically any version of *You are my good girl* or *Are you going to be my good girl?* works for me. I like to see it in writing so I can read it over and over again when I'm at work.

Sabrina, 33

She shoves her fingers in my mouth and pulls my hair by my ponytail while she tells me how naughty I've been. I'm naked on the chair, but she puts all of my clothes back on and tells me that I'm going to have to wait while she pulls something over my eyes so I cannot see a thing. She steps away and I can hear her fiddling with things—maybe her boots or maybe she is undressing or maybe she has something new for me. She's making noise, and I'm just waiting. I can hear her coming back toward me, and she puts her hand over my mouth and I can barely breathe. Then she shoves her whole hand in my mouth and tells me to suck it.

She continues with this for a while. Coming close, fiddling with my clothes and telling me I've been bad, and then walking away leaving me waiting . . .

Mara, 25

When she tells me that she loves me, I find it so sexy. And if she's touching me or kissing me and whispers that she loves me, I get so turned on.

Alex, 31

She travels for work, and on her way home last year, she sent me a photo of her fingers. They were shiny and wet and it said something like, "I'm all wet thinking about you. See you tonight." I've never been so turned on in my life. I guess it was the buildup, because I had to wait a few hours to see her and I thought I was going to explode.

Taylor, 34

He calls me at work and tells me he's thinking about me. He's not too explicit, but he tells me that he's getting hard just thinking of the last time we were together. He says he's *throbbing*. He says he cannot concentrate because the thought of my skin, my body, my touch is just too much. He whispers that I'm *intoxicating*. He says someone is coming and that he'll call me back. He calls me back an hour later apologizing and keeps telling me just how badly he wants me. It's like he has studied every inch of my body: *I want your lips. They are soft and warm. Your skin makes me want you—I want to smell and taste your cheeks, your neck, your spine, and work my way down.* He pauses between every line, waiting for me to react, but I say nothing. He's breathing so heavily. *I love your breasts. They are perfect. And god—your nipples.* He goes on awhile. And he keeps calling all day long. Laying it on thick every time. He texts me when he's leaving the office and again when he's in the car—like he's warning me that he's coming for me. He gets himself ready in the car so he can just walk in and take me. I do not have to do a thing, and he looks me up and down like it's the first time.

Jenni, 31

Seduction for me isn't sexual. It is really about being relaxed. I know other guys want their partners to drop to their knees as soon as they come home. That's my nightmare. I don't like the pressure. Seduction needs to build. I want to decompress. I want to talk about my day and hear about my partner's. I need time together to feel like we're connected. I tend to worry a lot, so if we chat about daily stuff, it puts my mind at ease. And then I need physical contact. Once we get into bed, I like a few minutes of just lying together. I'm always a little tense at first. It's not just about sex—I'm like that with everything. So I find that touching helps the tension to subside, and then I get in the mood. Once I'm in the mood, I do not mind taking the lead and doing whatever they are into.

Braeden, 27

I'm a very confident, intelligent alpha man. I become seduced and very submissive and sexual when a woman shows her intelligence. But even more sexy than that is her level of awareness. Some would label it sapiosexuality. I think my alpha monkey brain wants to create intelligent offspring. I wasn't always like this—I used to be intimidated and almost impotent when I was seduced by an intelligent and aware woman. I work hard to repair the mind vs. body split that I was trained to have. I use NLP and the study of self-esteem to be with the right kind of person (interested in reality) and to be sexually attracted to her at the same time. I'm very excited to be in my fifties and automatically attracted to the right kind of people for me.

Daniel, 50-something

I once had a girlfriend who was obsessed with food, and she was always using meals to seduce me. She'd cook me all these different dishes and then get up from the table to feed me a little. Sometimes the food was so good, and sometimes it was out of my comfort zone, but I just remember loving the enthusiasm she had for food and also for sex. Now that I'm dating again, I cannot help but assume that a woman who loves food will also love sex and let the passion transfer from one room to the other. Now I cook more, so I want the seduction to go both ways. I want a lover who will cook for me and feed me, and even do it right on the dinner table while the food is still there. And I want to do the same. I want a lover I can seduce with food. My ultimate seduction fantasy is cooking together and getting messy in the kitchen. I want to set a really nice table with fancy utensils, plates, and glassware and sit down to eat. But I want to feed her, and I want her to love the food so much that she begs for me to get down on my knees and eat her out right at the table.

Ashley, 45

When I ask my lover to put cream on my back, that's a sign that I'm in the mood. It doesn't mean I'm ready to start right that second, but once we start touching, I feel like sex is at least possible. But I do not like when they rub my back for a minute and then head straight for the reach around right away. I want a few minutes of just physical touch so I don't feel pressured. And then I'll return the favor. I actually really like massaging my lover's legs and eventually making my way in between them. That's my ultimate seduction.

Fatima, 25

I like when sex and seduction are intense. A little conflict gets me going, and I don't like gentle, tender sex as much as I like a challenge. You'll see it on TV, for example—couples who love-hate one another. That's my style. Of course in my relationships,

I want love, but I like to role-play a little tension. If I'm irritable or frustrated, I want my lover to use sex to assuage the discomfort. And I'm happy to work for it too, if that's what they're into.

Xie Xie, 27

We play a game where he pretends to pick me up on the street. He drives by in his car, and we pull off at the side of the road. He takes care of me first with his hands. If I'm up for it, I repay the favor, and then he just drops me home.

Leyla, 38

We're working from home, and we're overwhelmed with work. He's sitting across from me typing away, and I'm doing the same. We both look up and our eyes meet, and then we run upstairs to the bedroom and tear our own clothes off. It is quick and dirty, and we get right back to work after we're done.

Jennifer, 33

I like when my partner comes on to me when I'm busy. If I'm cooking dinner or on the phone, I want them to come over and get handsy with me. Being interrupted while doing something mundane is so hot.

Ananya, 44

Old-fashioned manners turn me on. If you want to seduce me, say *please* and *thank you* and throw in a *yes ma'am* or *as you wish* before we go up to bed. I know it is a bit of a role-play, but there is something about language that makes me weak in the knees.

Kristen, 53

Being seduced by a stranger is my ultimate fantasy. If my partner gives me some time to fantasize about it or even talks to me about this fantasy, that's the best thing he can do to seduce me. Tap into my seduction fantasy: I meet them at a party. Every time I look in their direction, it's clear that they are staring at me—enthralled. They smile and walk over. We chat for a few minutes, but it is clear that we only have one thing on our minds. We get split up and come back together several times over the course of the night, but I know they'll come find me before the night ends. It's almost time to go home, and they are following me around as I socialize. They take me by the hand and lead me into a closet or a bathroom or a bedroom (I do not really care). They take off their scarf or their tie and blindfold me before it all begins . . .

Tamara, 49

Dress up like a cowgirl. Or a nurse or a bunny or a clown. I don't really care. Any costume will do. I'm seduced by the creative, and I'm very visual. Once she dressed up like pumpkin for Halloween, and that did it for me too.

Paul, 54

SEDUCTION INSTRUCTION

What is your ultimate seduction fantasy? Can you write it down in point form, flesh it out in prose or poetry, or sketch a version of what you want?

Consider the following prompts to help guide you:

▸ Where does your seduction fantasy take place?

▸ Who is present for your seduction fantasy?

▸ What do you look like? What are you wearing?

▸ How are you feeling in your fantasy?

▸ What does your lover (or lovers) look like? What are they wearing?

▸ What sounds do you hear?

▸ What sights can you see?

▸ Are there any smells or tastes that play a role in this scene?

▸ What comes before your seduction fantasy?

▸ What follows?

▸ What are the tools that you need to implement your fantasy?

▸ What are the distractions that can get in the way, and how can you address them?

▸ What are some alternative ways you can complete your seduction fantasy without doing it all? Are there pieces of it that you can use in real life?

You don't have to answer all of these questions, and your seduction fantasies may range from one word to a thousand (or more). Some people fantasize vividly in great detail and specificity, and others find that their fantasies are more general and fleeting. However you fantasize, give yourself permission to explore uncharted territory and let your mind wander far from reality.

Continue to add to your fantasy as new ideas emerge, and don't worry if your thoughts do not make perfect sense or if an old fantasy tends to contradict a new one. Fantasies are often a mishmash of thoughts, dreams, memories, and desires, and they are constantly evolving.

Tap into Your Sexual Fantasies

If you have difficulty tapping into your seduction fantasies, look for other sources of inspiration. Ask you lover(s) and friends to share their stories and fantasies. Read erotic fiction or think about some of the ways you've responded to sex and seduction scenes you've read about in books or seen on screen. You may also want to consider if your beliefs or the feelings you associate with sex (e.g., shame) are stymieing your fantasies.

You need not feel guilty about your sexual fantasies—whatever they entail. Even if your fantasies fall outside the boundaries of your real-life relationships, they can improve the quality of your sex life and deepen connection. Not only do your fantasies help you to learn more about yourself (and your partner, if you share and discuss), but they also prime your body and mind for arousal. Most folks find that the more they fantasize, the more sex they desire.[2]

You will likely benefit from sharing your fantasies with your partner and encouraging them to do the same. This not only intensifies your connection, but the mere discussion of sex can also lead to arousal. You don't have to share every detail of every fantasy (you're allowed to have private thoughts that are just for you!), but if you can discuss the themes, settings, and feelings associated with your seduction fantasies, it can help your partner to better understand how to approach you when they are in the mood.

If sharing your seduction fantasies leads to feelings of tension or insecurity, that's okay too. Tension and insecurity occur in all relationships. It can be hard to accept that your partner fantasizes about people and scenarios that are beyond the scope of your relationship. But it is perfectly normal. Researchers at the University of Vermont discovered that 98 percent of men and 80 percent of women have fantasized about someone other than their current partner in the past few months.[3] These fantasies tend to increase over time, which makes sense, as we have a natural desire for novelty and often use sex as an escape from reality. It is important to remember that indulging in a specific fantasy does not mean that you have a desire to try it out in real life. This is what makes fantasies so powerful: they allow us to play alternative roles in make-believe worlds, and though we can get lost in the moment (if we want to), this does not interfere with our ability to differentiate between fantasy and reality.

If your partner is reticent to open up and share their fantasies, consider turning to popular culture as a source of inspiration and conversation. When you watch movies or television shows, ask them how they feel about a specific sex scene. Ask them if they like it, and probe a little deeper to understand why or why not. Most shows and movies depict sex via seduction, so you will likely encounter a variety of scenarios to discuss. Oftentimes it's easier to talk about other people's interactions (e.g., fictional or historical characters) before you start discussing your own feelings, desires, and fantasies.

SEDUCTION INSTRUCTION

If you're nervous or cannot find the words to describe your fantasies, turn to art as a means of communication. Draw the seduction scenes you would like to try and enjoy a good laugh trying to decipher the visual representation of one another's fantasies. Since laughter helps to ease tension, deepen connection, and lower inhibitions, this exercise offers a series of corollary benefits. Go ahead and get your crayons, pencils, or paint (or digital application if you are tech fancy) and bring your seduction fantasies to life through art.

Playing out your fantasies in small doses helps to keep sex exciting in long-term relationships. You might simply try on a new accent, role, location, prop, or scenario. You do not have to act out your fantasies in their entirety—choose one element and try it on for size.

For example, if you fantasize about spontaneous sex with a stranger in public, you might role-play one small element with your partner—after your regular date-night dinner at a restaurant, "bump into" one another at the bar, introduce yourselves, and then sneak off to your car (or a washroom stall, if they're private with locks) and make out. You don't have to go all the way in public, but experiment with pieces of your fantasy, bearing in mind that you can build on it the next time around.

Another option is to start with *talk* alone. While you are making out or having sex, whisper some teasing and vague one-liners in your partner's ear. For example, if they fantasize about having a threesome, whisper, *I want to share you*. If they fantasize about being ravenously desired, remind them, *Everyone wants a piece of this*. If you feel embarrassed, play loud music or porn in the background so that your voice is not the only sound they hear.

Note that you do not need to bring your fantasies to life in order to use them as a source of arousal, intimacy, and pleasure. You may want to simply *talk* about your fantasies. Sometimes fantasies are more powerful in your head than in real life.

SEDUCTION INSTRUCTION

Jot down your thoughts in response to the following questions in your journal:

▸ Think about a time when you were sexually smitten by someone. What is it that they did that made your heart skip a beat and your body ache with desire? How did you respond?

▸ What could have made the situation better?

▸ Why do you think you still remember it to this day? Can you recall the smallest details about the experience?

▸ Would you like to share this experience and your insights with your partner(s)?

YOUR LEARNING STYLE
AS YOUR SEDUCTION STYLE

Just as we naturally develop personalities and styles when it comes to seduction and sex, we also have a preference for *learning styles* in the sexual realm. Research suggests that we learn through three predominant means: sight, sound, and touch. You may be a visual learner, an auditory learner, or a kinesthetic or tactile learner. Of course, most of us learn via multiple styles, and these categories offer a limited scope, as some folks cannot see, hear, or touch. However, it can be helpful to approach seduction—for yourself and for your lover(s)—through the lens of seduction styles in reference to learning styles.

You may already be familiar with your own learning styles as well as your lovers'. If you are primarily a visual learner, you may be most responsive to visual cues like charts, graphs, photos, and the written word. You may remember faces, take notes, and make lists, and in the bedroom, you may be particularly responsive to watching the action unfold. If you are an auditory learner, you may be sensitive to sounds, you might find it useful to read out loud, and you may find it helpful to talk to yourself. When it comes to sex, you may like to make lots of noise and want your lover(s) to do the same. If you are a kinesthetic learner, you may like to move around while you learn, and you might notice that you prefer to get a big-picture view first (e.g., scan this entire book and chapter titles) before diving into the details. You likely crave more touch and might find the physical component of sex most alluring.

As you discover your own learning style and preferences, you can teach your lover(s) what works best for you so that they become better equipped to cater to your needs. As you better understand their seduction style and preferences, you can adjust your approach to incorporate their seduction style into your repertoire.

SEDUCTION INSTRUCTION

Are you familiar with your (nonsexual) learning style(s)? Most of us are a combination of all three, but you may favor one over the others. There are many quizzes online, including a fairly short option at HowToLearn. com, so take a moment to try one now.

Regardless of your lover's seduction learning style, you can entice and enchant them by planting a *sex seed*. Sex seeds are seductive clues about what is to come in a future sexual experience. They can be planted in the morning if you want to get busy at night or throughout the week before you meet. To plant effective seeds, consider which erotic activities appeal to your lover. Do they like romantic sex? Do they love to be filmed? Are they publicly experimental? Select an erotic activity that you can plan on your own and plant a sex seed to set the tone. For example, if your partner likes to be spanked, leave a spanking instrument in their car (paddle, wooden spoon from the kitchen, riding crop) or leave a photo of it in their briefcase. Leave them a note in their lunch bag or text them a photo of it in your hands. Throughout the day (or week), water the sex seed by leaving additional clues. This process can offer you a distraction to reduce stress and help you to weave eroticism throughout your day-to-day interactions.

We offer suggestions for learning-style specific seduction and sex seed planting below.

Visual Seduction

For visual learners, pleasure is all about the eyes and the imagination. Visual-linguistic learners may be more responsive to the written word, including flirtatious texts, love notes, and naughty stories, and those who favor a visual-spatial style may enjoy photos, video clips, and playful peep shows.

Consider the following strategies to be a skilled visual seducer for your lover:

Make lots of eye contact. Visual folks crave consistent, steady eye contact and gauge attraction and mood by the way you look at them. Weave it into your general interactions to stay connected—not just when sex is imminent, but throughout the day and week. Consider Tyra Banks's advice that models ought to "smize," or smile with their eyes; not only can you smile with your eyes, but you can convey lust, admiration, and desire to rouse interest, cultivate eroticism, and seduce a visual learner.

Clean up the clutter. Visual people are distracted by a busy sightline. Simply put, you cannot compete with piles of laundry or a messy room when you are with a visual learner, so limit the clutter and make sure that everything has its own dedicated place. This applies to sexts and video chats too; it will not matter how hot you look in a photo if they're distracted by an unmade bed in the background.

Tell stories rich in detail. Visual folks are daydreamers. Cater to these dreams by drawing out the details of your stories, sex dreams, and fantasies. Remember to mention the little things, including colors, perspectives, and anything that can be visually imagined. For example, over dinner or in a casual situation, discuss a recent sex dream or fantasy: *I had a fantasy of being on video with you. We bought this state-of-the-art video camera. We set it up next to the dresser facing the mirror, and you start by giving me a striptease. You let your hair down. You're wearing that bright-red blouse with the ruffles that I like, and as you striptease, you slowly reveal your tattoos button by button . . .* etc. Go into as much detail as possible.

Dress impeccably. This goes without saying, but visual people are a fan of anything that stands out. Depending on their taste, this might include tattoos, piercings, and eye-catching fashion. Bold choices and variety are likely to draw them in. Do you have a pair of heels that you can barely walk in, but they are amazingly sexy? Offer to wear them exclusively in the bedroom. Lay out sexy outfits on the bed so that they get a preview. Take them shopping and try on outrageous outfits even if you have nowhere to wear them.

Be the opposite of the room. Show up a little late to the party to make a grand entrance or be the opposite of the movement in the room. If the room is standing still (like a dinner party), move around to get their attention. If the room is busy (like a bar or club), stand still or move purposefully and slowly throughout the room.

For the visual lover, consider the following approaches to planting a sex seed:

▶ Send a sexy or naughty pic of yourself to their phone or personal (not work!) email.

▶ Send them sexy pics of other people (within the public domain—photos you are allowed to share) and ask them if they like it.

▶ Send a quick shot of a body part that is close-up or unclear so they have to fill in the blanks.

▶ Pull out your favorite toy and let them walk in while you are playing with yourself.

▶ Tell them about something that you saw that turned you on, and make sure that you share vivid details.

▶ Turn on a sexy video or porn and wait for them in bed.

▶ Straddle them facing in either direction so they get a beautiful view of your body.

▶ Do a slow striptease for them, removing layer after layer.

▶ Write them a playful note describing what you want to do to them later, or make a list of what makes them a great lover. Bonus points for legible writing!

Auditory Seduction

Sounds are essential to auditory learners, and their yearnings span beyond talking dirty and hearing you scream their name. Research suggests that the sound of a lover's voice can be a turn-on resulting in increased electrical activity in the skin.[4] And our voices may even indicate fertility due to hormonal fluctuations that affect blood flow and water retention in the vocal cords. Whether your lover is an auditory learner or a combination of multiple styles, consider these approaches to leave them singing your praises:

Give them feedback. People who learn from and respond to auditory cues often love to hear themselves speak. They love the sound of many voices—including their own—and want others to hear what they have to say. To seduce someone who loves to talk, be an active, present listener and ask them questions to win them over. Encouraging them to speak may seem counterintuitive (since they also like to listen), but you will be stroking their ego and fulfilling the universal desire to feel heard and valued.

Expand your vocabulary. When you vary your vocabulary or use language that is uncommon in everyday chatter, you arouse their interest. If they are not familiar with a term or phrase, they may be drawn in and become curious to uncover what else you have to share and teach. Taking your time to pronounce words with multiple syllables in a purposeful drawl can affect them in a similar way. You can even use words that you wouldn't use on an everyday basis. For example, if you are a squirter, mention that you cannot wait to experience the incomparable *amrita* the next time you spend time with them.

Use low, soft, deep tones. High-pitched sounds can be off-putting, and speaking slowly, emphatically, and calmly will leave them hanging off your every word. You might also vary your speed and cadence once in a while to maintain their interest, as they can be responsive to fluctuations in sounds. Those with experience in ASMR (autonomous sensory meridian response) know that the sound of a voice alone can create tingly associations in the head and neck as well as feelings of euphoria and pleasure.

Play their favorite music. Most of us are moved by the sound of music, but auditory learners are particularly sensitive and may find that specific vibrations and melodies can have a significant impact on their mood. Ask them what songs make them feel sexy, relaxed, or powerful and adjust your playlist accordingly.

Highlight your moans and breathy tones when you are intimate. Auditory people crave sound, and some feel uncomfortable with silence. If you are quiet in bed, consider learning to project your sounds and allow your breath to guide your body; this can draw their attention to the present moment and help them to be more mindful of the experience. Remember that we tend to gauge our lovers' arousal and pleasure levels based on their sounds and breath rates, so be effusive in your expressions and be sure to explore the section on dirty talk in the Verbal Seduction chapter.

Plant one of these sex seeds for your auditory lover:

▶ Text them sound clips of sex or sexy sounds. Bijoux Indiscrets has a library of sex sounds at orgasmsoundlibrary.com if you are not comfortable making your own.

▶ Whisper something simple in their ear in public or even at the dinner table. *You're so hot. I've been thinking about you all day.*

▶ Tell them that you see other people checking them out to play into the nearly universal desire to be desired.

▶ Record an audio clip of yourself masturbating (e.g., in the shower to muffle your sounds) and send them the file. Better yet, tell them all about it and make them wait for it.

▶ Read them a few lines from an erotic story—in person or

on the phone. You can also make a recording of an erotic story as a special treat.

▶ Leave them a note telling them what *you* want, or send them a voice note.

▶ Write *I want you* on the mirror while they're in the shower and then meet them in bed. (They can imagine the sound of your voice as they read your note.)

▶ Talk dirty and tell them all the thoughts you savor when you think about them.

Tactile Seduction

Kinesthetic learners are generally attracted to movement and touch. They may be easily distracted and lose interest if they are physically disconnected, and they often express love, desire, and affection through touch and want you to do the same. For many, tactile seduction is the most obvious approach to sex, but we often rush into the usual outcome-based routine rather than allowing the desire to mount and indulging in the process of seduction itself.

To build tension and desire with a tactile lover:

Use different points of pressure. Most people use their hands, but you can use any body part to vary the sensations and pressure. Using the palms of your hands or solid parts of your body to put a little pressure on your tactile person can be very seductive and make them feel safe and desired. For example, while watching a movie, put your leg on top of theirs so they can feel the warmth and weight of your body. Alternatively, tickle the sides of your hands down their neck when they are sitting at their desk to maintain the connection even when sex is off the table.

Dance with them! Not only does movement (e.g., dance, exercise, yoga) breed confidence, but as we learn to appreciate and trust in our body's performance, our connection to our physical self intensifies. Moreover, dancing builds physical endurance, coordination, flexibility, and strength—all of which come in handy when you are hanging off the chandelier or getting creative between the sheets. You don't have to be a great dancer to press your body against your lover's and sway to the bass (or the treble) of your favorite song. Lean into their hips, tenderly curl your hands around their neck, or turn down the lights to perform a lap dance to leave them eating out of the palm of your hand.

Play with fabric. Most of your clothes may be made of cotton, but tactile lovers are attracted to texture. Look for scarves, stockings, sweaters, and sheets that will make them want to touch you the same way they like to touch clothes on the rack in the store. To enhance the sense of touch when you are in the bedroom, blindfold your lover(s) and use anything from fur and feathers to satin and/or silk to stimulate the nerves on their skin.

Use *their* hands. Take them by the hand and show them how to touch you. They find your touch alluring, but tactile lovers also love to feel your body with their own hands. Run their hands over your butt at breakfast, take them by the hand on the car ride home, or wrap their arms right around you while you are snuggling on the couch. And consider other body parts too. They'll be open to following your lead and will likely be overrun with desire if you simply press your naked body against theirs—in bed, in the shower, or anywhere else you can get away with being naked.

Use push and pull movements. When pushed or pulled, it is natural to pull or push in response, as the body cannot help but rebel. But if you push your lover first and then pull away (create opposing sensations), it comes as a surprise and can pique their interest. For example, gently push their hips away from you and then pull them toward you. You can do this with various body parts, including the neck, head, or shoulders, to experiment with dominance, submission and switching roles.

Sex seed suggestions for the tactile/kinesthetic:

▶ Wiggle your way into them as the big or small spoon and cuddle while they are reading or watching a show.

▶ Send them videos that depict touching: lick your lips, run your fingertips over your lips, cup your breasts, rub your chest over your clothes, or gently rub your hand against your thigh. These clips do not have to be clear or perfect. In fact a shaky hand can be even more beguiling, as they are forced to try to decipher the images.

▶ Slip them the tongue when they are just expecting a peck, and then lock eyes for a moment before you walk away and leave them wanting more.

▶ Tease them when they are busy. Fondle them for just a few seconds while they're on a call or give them a naughty squeeze before they walk out the door.

▶ Give them a one-minute massage (hand, scalp, calves, feet, or shoulders) to start their day, and feel free to do it in the nude.

▶ Run your thumb delicately over their lips after your kiss.

▶ Dance naked with them.

SEDUCTION INSTRUCTION

Have your lover take the seduction quiz to better understand how they want to be seduced. Plan a carefully thought-out date (or mini date) that caters to their seduction learning style and solicit feedback during the experience. You can find the seduction learning style quiz here: http://bit.ly/VLQuiz1

Tap into Your Other Senses

Tuning into your senses is one of the most effective ways to explore seduction. It helps you to be more present and feel the full experience within your entire body. Your sense of touch is almost always heightened during sexual seduction and arousal, but your other senses can be equally powerful. Your sense of smell, for example, can help you to gauge compatibility with a potential partner, and your sense of taste has the potential to rile you up, but also to quash all sexual desire.

Olfactory Seduction

Smell is biological, and evolutionary theories suggest that we use it to assess mate compatibility. For example, if you find someone's natural scent (without the interference of deodorants, perfumes, etc.) repulsive, you may have similar immune markers, which indicates that you should not procreate together. This theory, however, reflects cisgender heterosexual interactions and may not apply given the range of relationships we engage in and the technological advances in reproductive technology.

But smells also seal our fondest (and most repulsive) memories, and sexual response is affected by scents, so the olfactory system plays a role in seduction regardless of gender identity and sexual orientation. You can use scent to attract and seduce lovers in several ways:

Cook for them. Most people love to smell food, which is why chocolate chip cookie candles and pumpkin spice everything sell like hotcakes—and do not get us on started on the delicious smell of hotcakes. When you cook for your partner, not only is this a generous act of service (one of Gary Chapman's five love languages), but you both benefit from the mood boost and the creation of a positive memory. Ask your lover to describe their favorite meal of all time and try to recreate it together or as a surprise.

Light scented candles or incense. Identify their preferences by asking them what smells they like and recall fondly. Do they like the scent of fresh linen or clothes coming out the dryer? Do they love the smell of the ocean? Are they a fan of strong scents or subtle ones? Get to know their preferences and consider some research findings suggesting that specific scents may aid in arousal; one study found that combining scents like pumpkin, lavender, licorice, and even doughnuts can increase penile blood flow, and though this is only one measure of arousal, circulation plays a significant role in sexual arousal and response.[5]

Attract them with body scents—perfumes, colognes, body sprays, or your natural odor. The initial scents that spark attraction are generally the scents that sustain it over time. For example, if you wore a specific perfume when you first met, it may always remind your lover of your body—even when others wear the same scent. It can also encourage them to subconsciously recall fond memories from the early stage of your relationship to reinvigorate feelings of passion.

Because familiarity can breed comfort and desire, your natural body scent can become even more appealing as your lover becomes accustomed to it over time; research suggests that no two people interpret smells in the same way, which is part of why smell preferences are highly personal.

Note: if you have a new partner, be sure to ask them about their scent tolerance to be mindful of scent sensitivities.

Gustatory Seduction

Seducing someone via taste is a unique experience, and the desire for food often mirrors the desire for sex. Food and sex both elicit a sensory response, and our experiences of these pleasures are affected by what we see, hear, feel, taste, and smell. Just as we can be turned on and off by the smell and taste of foods, so too are we affected by the scent and taste of a partner.

When considering gustatory seduction, consider **oral hygiene first.** Take good care of your mouth by flossing, brushing your teeth, using mouthwash, and regularly seeing your dentist (if you can). Bad breath ranks as a near-universal turnoff, so taking care of your oral health lays the groundwork for oral interactions from kissing to going down. Before you kiss, ensure that you like the taste of your own mouth, and rinse with water if you do not have anything else on hand, as you may not be able to smell your own breath.

Include taste in your quest to seduce, and appeal to your partner's palate by cooking foods that are associated with heightened libido, sexual functioning, and overall health. Some foods that may positively affect your sex life include **oysters**, **whole grains**, **legumes**, and **seafood**, which are high in zinc; **soy milk** and **coconut milk**, which are vitamin-D fortified; and

cherries, which are a source of melatonin, the hormone that helps to regulate the circadian rhythm and promote a good night's sleep.

Food lovers are also generally responsive to surprise treats, so stock your pantry or handbag with snacks to stave off their hunger and support libido. **Pumpkin seeds** are high in zinc, vitamins, and minerals, and they contain tryptophan, which can promote serotonin production to boost mood. **Blueberries** are rich in flavonoids, which are considered antioxidants; **maca** is believed to support the adrenal glands, which work overtime in response to stress; and **nuts** contain omega-3 fatty acids and L-arginine, which are linked with nitrous oxide to fuel strong erectile functioning.

There is no magic bullet or sexual superfood, but healthy eating affects your mood, energy levels, sleep patterns, and cardiovascular health—all of which interact with sexual desire and response.

If you want to improve the way you eat, **make small changes to your diet**, acknowledging that you do not need to overhaul it overnight. Research and choose two to three healthier foods you would like to eat together and consider cutting one undesirable habit at a time. (You know your body best, so do not let others dictate what is healthy, especially if their standard of health has to do with a narrow version of weight or beauty.) You might add berries and nuts to your morning cereal or opt for a side of vegetables instead of fries at lunch twice a week. You might cut back on chicken wings by one piece per meal or refrain from drinking soda pop three days per week. Small changes to your diet can amount to more significant results than massive over-hauls, as you are more likely to follow through and maintain these habits in the long run.

Consuming healthier foods not only affects your emotional and physical health, but your diet can affect the scents you naturally exude and the way your genitals taste. We do not have scientific data to confirm the link between diet and genital taste, but supertasters (e.g., adult film stars who consider themselves orally experienced) have observed that diets high in fruits and vegetables produce sweeter tastes, and fried and processed foods result in more bitter flavors.

In addition to considering how the foods you consume affect your sex life, **you may also want to play with food with your lover**. Your options are endless, so experiment and enjoy the process even if each new approach is not a grand slam. Freeze grapes and pop them into your mouth during oral sex. Lick honey off their nipples. Paint chocolate over their chest. Use cinnamon to create a tingly sensation across their skin. Feed them strawberries with your fingers. Give them a champagne blow job or massage. Decorate cupcakes together in the nude. You might find that connecting food with sexual seduction encourages you to approach both eating and sexual activity more mindfully.

Though you may not include all five senses in every seduction routine, try to consider the ways in which your lover responds to sensory seduction and highlight those that are most appealing to them. Be creative and be sure to change things up, as variety and unpredictability make you more attractive and increase the chances of your lover responding favorably to your seductive advances in the long run.

SEDUCTIVE COMMUNICATION: CONVERSATIONS FOR HOTTER SEX

Talking about sex can be just as exciting and arousing as having sex. But it can also be intimidating. Despite the fact that we are surrounded by depictions of sex and sexual messages, these popular portrayals are often at odds with our own desires and lived experiences.

The bodies, positions, interactions, and responses you see in porn, for example, may not reflect the types of sex you genuinely desire; similarly the storylines, relationships, and connections depicted in rom-coms are unlikely to mirror those you've encountered in real life. If you are a person of color, queer, kinky, consensually nonmonogamous, a person with a disability, older, and/or fat, your experiences with sex and relationships are even less likely to be acknowledged and celebrated in popular media. **It follows that we have to unlearn commonly accepted sexual stereotypes (and help our partners to do the same).**

This is why *talking* about sex is essential. Communication is not only a form of seduction (we'll get to this very soon, we promise!), but a precursor that lays the foundation for more meaningful, fulfilling, and pleasurable sex.

If, however, you are uncomfortable talking about sex with

your lover, know that you are not alone. Without exception, we all struggle to communicate our needs, boundaries, preferences, and desires at times. No matter how confident you are, sex can be a challenging topic to address, as it is both highly personal and socially stigmatized. It intersects with so many other components of our identities, from the political and personal to the social and physical. Even as so-called experts in the field, we sometimes find ourselves at a loss for words in our personal relationships. But we know we need to push through the discomfort, as these intense conversations are invaluable. They not only have the potential to heighten intimacy and pleasure, but they also improve the overall quality of relationships.

If you are struggling to start a conversation about sex or feel uncomfortable asking for what you want, consider this three-part approach that you can adjust to suit your needs.

- ▶ Highlight the positive.
- ▶ Ask questions and/or make an offer.
- ▶ Make your request.

Highlight the positive and begin with lighter topics. Start by talking about what you already enjoy about your sex life, and offer genuine compliments whenever possible. This initial conversation doesn't need to lead immediately to requests and critiques and it is not a one-shot deal. You can break the discussions up over the course of several days or weeks so that sex-related communication becomes the norm. Ideally, your comfort levels will increase, and sex talk will become a regular part of your interactions, as opposed to awkward discussions you have when you encounter problems in your sex life. By regularly acknowledging and appreciating the positive elements of your sex life, you normalize sexual conversations as constructive and ongoing, as opposed to reactionary.

Here are a few lines to get you started with positive sex talk:

I really love when you . . .
You are the best at . . .
I'll never forget how you . . .
One thing that I really like is . . .
Do you remember that time when you . . . ? That felt so good!
The most charming thing you do is . . .
Your _____ is nothing but perfect.
You are the greatest when you . . .
I genuinely love your approach to . . .

Asking questions to learn more about your lover's needs and feelings also improves sexual understanding, communication, pleasure, and seduction. No person is a universally great lover, but a willingness to listen and learn goes a long way.

With most skill-based activities, we receive formal instruction from our parents, teachers, experts, and peers. This learning might include courses, demonstrations, videos, formal practice, evaluation, and ongoing feedback. Sex, however, is an exception. We are expected to engage in hot, fulfilling sex without any formal education and with very few (if any) opportunities for observation.

Most of us have never had the opportunity to watch live, unscripted sex, so we make assumptions about what our partners want based on what we've seen in porn. But porn is primarily intended to entertain and titillate and is not produced with educational outcomes in mind. Just as you cannot learn to drive from watching NASCAR or *The Fast and the Furious*, you will not learn about the diversity and nuances of sex from porn. And you certainly will not learn about what your partner wants unless you ask them.

Some questions to start or continue your sexual conversation might include:

> *Do you like when I . . . ?*
> *Show me how you like it in this position . . .*
> *What can I do for you right now?*
> *What did you think about that scene in a film or TV show we watched together?*
> *If I were to seduce you tomorrow, what would you want me to do?*
> *Is there anything you would like me to do to make sex more enjoyable for you?*
> *Where do you like to be touched?*
> *What words do you want me to use/avoid?*
> *After you climax, how do you want to be touched/held?*
> *What would you like to do after we have sex?*

Making offers and acknowledging that you're willing to consider feedback and make adaptations to meet your partner's needs can increase the likelihood that they'll want to do the same. When you admit that you don't know it all, your partner is likely to follow suit, and expressions of vulnerability—of any kind—tend to bring you closer together.

Sex talk will be easier and more fruitful if it's a two-way exchange, as opposed to a one-directional lecture. If you are more naturally inclined toward verbal expression than your partner, take a step back and encourage them to open up so the conversations are not one-sided. Listen intently and ask for clarification as needed. Look to yourself first to identify opportunities for growth, rather than asking your partner to change to meet your needs; *you will get more of what you want if you focus on what you are willing to give first.*

Making requests and setting boundaries will become easier as you become accustomed to highlighting the positive and asking questions, and your comfort level talking about sex will likely increase. Expressing your desires and interests with care and tact can be a challenge, and you can expect your lover to be sensitive to your speech, tone, and body language. If your lover becomes defensive when you make a request, offer reassurance that your requests do not reflect a deficit, but are an indication of your love, commitment, and attraction. You may want to encourage your lover to share their requests first so that you can model receptiveness to their needs.

And always consider how your approach affects your partner's response. Are you really making a *request* or are you lodging a *complaint*? Have you considered how you can make changes (cognitive or behavioral) to meet your own needs first or have you placed the onus of responsibility on your partner alone? Do you balance requests with positive reinforcement and do you ensure that incidents of the latter far outweigh the former? Oftentimes, we become frustrated with our partner's reactions to our requests without considering how our approach contributed to eliciting their reaction. So if you want something from your partner, ensure that your request isn't really a veiled complaint or criticism. You have a right to ask for what you want, but you want to be mindful of your partner's feelings too.

Consider trying these conversation starters when making sexual requests:

I would love more _____. You are so good at it.

I had a dream about trying _____ with you, and it got me thinking . . .

I read an article about _____. What do you think of that?

I have the best orgasms when you _____.

*In an ideal world, I'd like to have sex (however you define it) X
times per week. What can we do to make more time/find a
balance?*

One thing I'd like to work on is . . .

*I would like to explore this type of fantasy. Are you open to that?
Why or why not?*

Talking about sex isn't a one-shot deal. It is an ongoing conversation that can include laughter, tension, and awkward moments. It is the tension and awkwardness that will only intensify passion and attraction later on. So relax, take a deep breath, and start talking! You will be glad you did.

SEDUCTION INSTRUCTION

Fill out the following questionnaire on your own in your journal. Notice how you respond to the questions when you read them for the first time. Have you considered these questions in the past, and why might you have avoided them?

Set a reminder in your calendar to revisit your notes in three months, six months, and/or one year. Consider why things have changed over time. Why do you think your answers might be the same or different? Are there any new sexual fantasies that have arisen? Our bodies, feelings, and ideas change over time, so it can be helpful to come back to this questionnaire every once in a while to reevaluate.

Self-Questionnaire:

▶ Do you remember the very first time you talked about sex with a partner? How have you changed and grown since that conversation?

▶ When did you last start a conversation about sex? How did you initiate the discussion and what might you do differently?

▶ Can you recall a time your partner(s) talked to you about sex? How did you respond? If you could go back in time, how would you adjust your response?

▶ When do you usually talk about sex? Is there a time that might work better?

▶ Where do you usually talk about sex? Is there a place that might work better?

▶ What makes talking about sex easier?

▶ What holds you back from opening up about sex?

▶ If you could ask your partner(s) one thing related to sex, what would it be?

▶ What could you do differently to enhance your sex life?

Talking About Sexual Frequency

One of the most important conversations you will have with regard to sex pertains to sexual frequency. Understanding your partner's preferences with regard to frequency will help you gauge how and when to seduce them.

And though quality is likely more important than quantity, sexual frequency and discrepancies in desire are significant and common sources of friction in relationships, so we want you to talk about it—even if it's not an issue at this time.

You cannot expect your desire for sex to perfectly align with your partner's over the course of many years or a lifetime. That would be like asking them to want the same foods in the same quantity at the same time every day for the rest of your lives. It is not realistic.

SEDUCTION INSTRUCTION

Part I: The Frequency Exercise

Talk about sexual frequency—in hard numbers. Even though your desire for sex fluctuates, it is essential to be specific about how often you would like to have sex. Do you want it once a day, once a week, or once a quarter? Oftentimes, we think we know how often our partner wants it, but we are not accurate at estimating their needs.

If you want sex less often than your partner, it is likely that you *overestimate* how often they want it, because it feels like they're always asking for it.

If you want sex more often than your partner does,

it is likely that you *underestimate* how often they want it, because it feels as though they're never interested or always saying no.

By formalizing the conversation, you will improve understanding and be better equipped to find common ground and meet one another's needs.

Get started now:

▶ Write down how often you want to have sex on a piece of paper. Do you want it once per week, once per hour, or once per fiscal year? Be honest. You are allowed to want it every day, and you are also allowed to not want sex at all. Draw a line below your number.

▶ Below the line, write down how often you believe your partner wants to have sex. Do you think they want it once per day, once per month, or once with every meal?

▶ Share your papers, have a laugh, and then have a discussion about how you can find some middle ground.

You might be on the same page as your partner, and you might feel as though you're still a world apart— either experience is okay. You can cultivate compatibility if you are both willing to put in the effort.

Part II: Lovers' Inquiry— Sexual Accelerants and Impediments

To better understand your own needs with regard to

sexual frequency and your partner's, **make a list of things that increase your desire for sex (accelerants) as well as a list of things that decrease your desire for sex (impediments)**. Consider experiences, interactions, feelings, and behaviors—both internal (related to yourself), external (related to life in general), and relational (related to your partner).

For example, perhaps you are more interested in sex when you exercise, dance, cook at home, get a good night's rest, spend time alone, read a book, listen to a specific song, finish the laundry, wake up early, stay up late, stand up for yourself, or enjoy a glass of tea. Or perhaps you find you want sex more frequently when you kiss, cuddle, read together, share a bath, laugh, take a break from chores, fantasize, eat candy, or decorate your room with flowers from the garden. These are some of your sexual seduction accelerants.

On the flip side, you might find that your interest in sex decreases when you watch the news, scroll on social media, play with your kids, talk to your roommate, eat a heavy meal, or work late. You might also lose interest when your partner works late, you eat dinner separately, or you talk about money. These are examples of your sexual seduction impediments.

These are just a few examples. The possibilities are endless and no two people will share the same lists.

Discuss your list with your partner, and become familiar with theirs to help you better understand how to meet one another's needs. Ask questions for clarification, look for overlaps, and devise strategies to find common ground. The Frequency Exercise and the Sexual Accelerants and Impediments inquiry are designed to help you start the conversation that will make space for finding common ground. You may also want to consider:

▸ Alternative activities in which to engage when one partner is in the mood and the other is not (e.g., toys, self-pleasure, other forms of intimate connection, lending a hand, exploring ways to get in the mood).

▸ Lifestyle changes to adjust your desire for sex (e.g., exercise, mindfulness, meditation, positive self-talk, fantasizing, masturbation) if you want to want more sex.

▸ Strategies and support your partner can offer to encourage interest in sex (e.g., share workload, increase affection, spend quality time, eroticize daily interactions, improve sexual technique and seduction).

▸ Specific ways to indicate to one another that you're (not) in the mood so that you remain connected even when you're not having frequent sex—however you define it.

Remember that frequency only matters as much as *you* feel it matters. You do not need to have more or less sex unless you and/or your partner *want* to have more or less sex. You can have sex once a day and be satisfied, and you can have sex once a year (or not at all) and be fulfilled. It is a matter of determining how often you want it and finding a balance between your desired frequency and your partner's.

Your levels of desire for sex will fluctuate with time, so even if you are aligned today, you will want to repeat this exercise at regular intervals. Of course, you'll be better off if you focus on the quality of your sexual relationship as opposed to the frequency with which you have sex; however, because sexual and relational satisfaction are tied to sexual frequency, the better you understand your partner's expectations, the better lover you will be when it comes to seduction, foreplay, and all types of sex.

VERBAL SEDUCTION

Your Own Kind of Dirty Talk

Talking about sex is not only a preamble to better sex, but also an effective approach to sexual seduction. Research suggests that when you talk about sex *during* sex, you experience higher levels of sexual self-esteem and satisfaction.[6]

Learning to seduce with your words is a skill that will enhance your sex life and may also improve overall communication. And learning to talk dirty can make sex more compelling and intense, as it engages multiple regions of the brain, including those involved in processing sound and emotion. This mind-body experience can be overwhelming and encourage you to use sex as an escape from reality.

But the term *dirty* is a bit of a misnomer, as dirty talk can make sex sweet, loving, raw, raunchy, edgy, fun, hot, and even funny. It need not be *dirty* in a pejorative or perverted sense— unless you want it to be!

With your words, you can bring fantasy to life and ensure that you get more of what you desire in bed (or in the back seat of your car). You can gab your way through fantasies and bring them to life in words alone. You can weave stories, play roles, switch personalities, make empty promises that feel real (with consent), and lead your lover into far off sexual and emotional lands that allow them to escape from mundane reality.

If you find dirty talk challenging or embarrassing, remember that you do not have to conform to any specific standard of *dirty*. For example, in porn, there tends to be an emphasis on screwing harder, faster, stronger, putting things in holes, getting rough, talking about size, and declaring a specific type of pleasure (e.g., *I'm coming!*). These approaches work for some people, but if they do not work for you, you can still embrace talking dirty in your own style.

For example, perhaps you are most turned on by monogamous romance. If this is the case, consider desirous dirty talk:

> *I'll never want anyone but you. You are too good and no one could ever compare.*
> *I love you so much. And when you do me like this, my love only deepens.*
> *I want this to last forever. I cannot imagine it any other way.*
> *Use me as your toy. I want to be yours all night long.*
> *You are mine. I adore how naughty you are.*
> *You are the only one for me. You can do anything with my body.*
> *I love how you treat me like a queen/king/royalty.*

Or perhaps you want to contemplate your consensually nonmonogamous fantasies or desires through dirty talk:

> *I cannot wait to share you.*
> *I'm ready for that threesome now.*
> *You deserve more than one lover, and I want to give it to you.*
> *I want to arrange the best orgy you've ever had.*

This weekend is all about you. They will all be here to please you.
Of course I want to share you. I've invited a friend over to play.

On the other hand, if you are turned on by sexual taboos, you might try some of these lines to get started:

Can you tie me up? It's something I've been wanting to experience.
I would love to give you a golden shower and get dirty with you.
I'd like to be your sexy kitten/perfect pup. Will you collar me?
Let's make porn together. I'd love to savor you on video.
I want to make love to you in public. Let's go to a sex club and
*   show off.*
Hold me down. I've been bad, and I want you to punish me with
*   your bare hands.*
Call me your daddy/mommy and beg me to spank you.

For those who like to tease and be playful, consider the following:

Do you like it when I touch you here? I like to wrap my hands
*   around you right there . . .*
I always get what I want. Remember that.
What a sweet, sexy butt you have . . .
You can have me any way you want . . .
Let's wrestle! Winner takes all . . .
You want this—don't you?
I know what you're thinking . . .

And if you like being dominant, play with these phrases and make them your own:

Babe, you have to follow all my rules right now.
Get on your hands and knees and wait like a good girl/boy.
Spread your legs wide for me. Your body is mine tonight.

You had better do what I say, or you will suffer the consequences.
I'm the boss! You will succumb to my desires.
Be good and fetch me my boots.
Do what I say or I won't let you come. But if you're good, I'll suck it all out with my lips.

On the flip side, perhaps you prefer to experiment with submission:

Maybe you should spank me. I've been very, very bad . . .
Get over here and show me who's boss!
Yes ma'am/sir, you can do whatever you like.
I am only here to fulfill your fantasies. Tell me what to do.
In your presence, I'm surrendering all my power to you.
I'm yours for the taking. Do as you wish.

If you simply want to use dirty talk to give directions, here are a few lines to get you started:

Come in my mouth. I want your taste on my tongue.
If that's what you want, grab my head and force me!
Do you love my juicy pussy/big dick? Tell me that you love it.
I want you to undress and wait for me in the bedroom.
Kiss me. I want more of you.
Tear my clothes off and have your way with me.
Get on your knees and shove your whole face in me.
Peel my clothes off slowly, one piece at a time.

Dirty talk can be used to cultivate consent:

Would you like to get nasty tonight?
Can I touch you in your naughty places?
What parts would you like my tongue to taste?

I'd love to put my fingers in _____. Will you let me?
I'd love to rub my [genitals] on your _____. Can I?
Can I tear your clothes off? It's all I've been thinking about.
Can I do you right here and toss you around like a rag doll?
Do you want me to hold you down while you scream and resist?
   (Use our safe word, "popcorn," if you want me to stop.)

And because seduction involves asking for what you want, you might use direct talk to make requests:

I want you to bend me over and make me scream . . .
Push your ass back toward me. I want to feel all of you.
I want you deeper inside me. Fill me up.
Come put your [genitals] in my mouth.
Put your mouth around my nipples and suck them hard.
I'm dying for you to wrap your lips around me.
I'm aching to feel your finger inside me while you kneel at my feet.
I want you to lie on the kitchen table and let me use all of my toys
   on you.

Oftentimes, we use dirty talk to live out our fantasies in a role-play or imaginative fashion:

You haven't been performing well on the court. It's time that I give
   you a private lesson.
You just broke the law. How are you going to fix it? Let's work
   something out.
I've never done this before. I mean, we just met.
What's your name again?
How much for the whole night? Whatever the cost, I know you're
   worth it.
My wife left for the weekend with the kids. Would you like to come
   over for dinner and a movie and . . . ?

> *You haven't been getting good grades. I'm going to give you some private tutoring.*
>
> *It sounds like your drain is plugged. I'll come over and clear the pipes for you. I'm good with my hands, and you can pay me back by stripping down and letting me touch.*

You can also consider using dirty talk to simply describe what you're doing, what you are about to do, or how you are feeling in the moment. This can be particularly useful if your partner cannot see what you're doing, or if you are seeking to build anticipation:

> *I'm going to get down on my knees. Do you like that?*
>
> *I'm stripping down, but I'm going to take my time. Do you want to watch, or should I just describe how I look?*
>
> *I've never felt so good. Keep filling me up. I can't get enough.*
>
> *I can feel your nipples getting hard. I cannot wait to get them between my teeth.*
>
> *I can feel myself getting wet. It's dripping down my thighs. Can you feel it too? I'm going to let you taste it on my fingers.*
>
> *I'm unlacing my boots, but I'll be a while. You're going to have to wait. You know it's worth it.*

And of course, you can utilize dirty talk to let your partner know just how great they are. Almost everyone is turned on by ego stroking, so lay it on thick and do not hold back if you are wild about your lover:

> *You are so fine. I just want to taste you and show you off to the world.*
>
> *I've never had it so good, and you make me want more and more. I'll never get enough of you.*
>
> *I come harder with you than I ever could have imagined. I can't take care of myself the way you do.*

I'd do anything to get more of you. I tell all my friends how lucky I am.

You taste so good. I crave you all day long.

Anyone would be lucky to have you. I can barely walk when we're done.

You're all I think about. I can't get any work done when I think of your naked body and the magic you work with those fingers and lips.

Some folks also find they are most turned on by recalling sexual memories—their sexual highlight reels—so you can also use dirty talk to seduce your lover with reference to the past:

Remember that time on the beach when . . .

I want to go back to that movie theater where we snuck into the back row . . .

Last night was so good. I can't stop thinking about the way you . . .

Remember when we watched that couple screwing around in the hammock . . .

Finally, you can use dirty talk in the future tense to seduce your lover via text, on the phone, through love notes, or by sending voice notes throughout the day:

When I get home, I'm going to throw myself between your legs, and I won't come up until you've gotten everything you could possibly desire.

Text #1: Want to hang tonight? Text #2: Naked?

When you come home, I'll have something waiting for you. And you won't be able to resist.

Let's skip the party and roll around on the living room floor. I want to taste you.

I'm going to tie you up and strip for you tonight. I'll make you wait for it, but it will be worth it.

I can't stop thinking about our bodies intertwined. What time can you meet so I can get my fix?

If you're new to talking dirty, simply begin with a word or two to let your lover know how you're feeling. *Yesss. Mmm. Ahh. Do not stop.* These simple words go a long way to provide generous but honest feedback. Let out a few moans, groans, and wide-mouthed exhales to indicate your pleasure. Allow the tension to mount gradually and start quietly, allowing your volume to increase with time.

Asking questions to encourage your lover to speak up is another simple approach to dirty talk. *Do you like that? Do you want me to make you come? Do you want me to come for you? Do you want it all over you? Do you want to taste me? Tell me how you like it. What can I do for you? I'll do anything . . .*

You might also find that you are more comfortable with dirty talk if you keep your volume low or your sounds muffled. For example, you might whisper in their ear or place a sheet over your mouth while you try out a few new lines. If you are on the phone, you can stifle your sounds with your hand over the receiver, and if you are video chatting, turn the lights down low and dampen your sounds if you are feeling shy. It can be hot to keep them guessing.

Sometimes you will misspeak, and sometimes the awkwardness will make you giggle, and that's okay. Laughter can help to cut the tension and bring you back to the present moment. Sex need not be serious, so relax and have a good time knowing that if something doesn't work out, you can try again tomorrow or next week.

Remember that one person's dirty talk is another's dinner conversation, so do not assume that what works for you will work for your lover(s).

As with all sex acts, if you want to use dirty talk to seduce your partner, you will need to ask them what they like. What words turn them on? What words are off-putting or upsetting? If your lover has survived (sexual) trauma, they may find certain words, phrases, or tones upsetting, so discuss these sensitivities and revisit this discussion often, as our preferences and comfort zones can change over time.

SEDUCTION INSTRUCTION

If you are still feeling nervous about talking dirty, remember that you don't have to do everything at once. In fact, you can practice your dirty talk in the comfort of your own home, in the car, or while riding your bike to work. Start by selecting three phrases from the lists above or come up with your own. Practice each phrase by repeating it over and over again with different inflections and emphasizing different words in the sentence. For example, the phrase "would you like to get nasty tonight?" can be uttered in a few different ways:

▸ Would YOU like to get nasty tonight?

▸ Would you like to get NASTY tonight?

▸ Would you like to get nasty TONIGHT?

Practice in different tones of voice and at different volumes to help you to find your rhythm. Repeating a phrase over and over again will help it to flow more naturally and will put you at ease when you utter it in the heat of the moment.

Nonverbal Seduction

Flirting is both an art and an evolutionary component that appears across all cultures. We use nonverbal flirtation and seduction to communicate desire in more diverse and nuanced ways. Rather than saying, "I'm interested in dating and/or having sex with you, and I'm wondering if the desire is mutual," we convey our interest with our body language, facial expressions, and hand gestures. These sometimes subtle and sometimes obvious cues allow us to test the waters and add variety to the way we approach potential partners and long-term lovers.

Nonverbal flirtation tends to be more common at the beginning of a relationship, and then it tapers off as we turn to words as our primary means of communication. But while "Are you in the mood?" is a perfectly acceptable approach to seduction, most of us are drawn in by an array of approaches—including playful signals that arouse our interest with an air of mystery.

If you want to flirt with and seduce your lover with your body, consider the following strategies:

▸ Brush up against them seductively when out in public. Run your hands over their thighs when you kiss goodbye or grab their butt while passing them in the kitchen.

▸ Smile whenever you make eye contact. You can smile for a moment and then look away, or gaze into their eyes with your lips wide.

▸ Touch their lower arm seductively with the backs of your fingertips; some theories suggest that the upper arm represents the friend zone and the lower arm is reserved for more intimate partners.

▸ Use a code word or signal to reference a sexual memory you share.

▸ Send sexy or flirtatious texts when they are sitting right next to you in a group. Whether you are out for dinner with friends or colleagues, remind them that you are thinking of them and that you are connected more intimately to one another than to anyone else at the table.

▸ Press up against them from behind whenever you have the chance. If you're reaching for a cup or leaning over to grab the remote, allow your bodies to connect for a few extra seconds.

▸ Look them up and down to show admiration. Lower your head and look up into their eyes before smiling and looking down.

▸ Sniff them! Lean in and inhale slowly and enthusiastically so they know you take comfort in their scent and thoroughly enjoy their body.

▸ Make eye contact at unexpected times. Sit across from one another at a party or gathering and sneak a coy smile as you lower your eyes.

▸ Turn your body toward them when you greet them. Stop what you are doing, smile, and touch their face or hands to connect.

▸ When you're waiting for them to get into bed, put down your book or phone and smile when they arrive. Wrap your legs around them to pull them close.

EMOTIONAL SEDUCTION
AND FOREPLAY

Seduction isn't just about what you say and do. **Ultimately, how your partner responds to you is a matter of how they *feel*.** And while you cannot control and you are not responsible for their emotions, you likely have a significant influence on how they feel about sex.

▶ When you approach them, do you make them feel *sexy*?

▶ When you look at them, do you make them feel *desired*?

▶ When you touch them, do you make them feel *loved*?

▶ When you kiss them, do you make them feel *playful*?

▶ Do your words evoke feelings of *shyness*, *playfulness*, *nervousness*, and/or *safety*?

▶ Do your actions lead to feelings of *power*, *subjugation*, *love*, and/or *relaxation*?

▶ Does your body language put them at ease and help them to *destress*?

▸ Does your language help them to feel *confident* and *empowered*?

▸ Does your approach make them feel safe being *vulnerable*?

▸ When you initiate sex, do they feel *surprised* and *excited*?

▸ Does spending time together make them *happy*?

The way you feel about sex is highly individual. And the feelings you associate with sexual desire, arousal, pleasure, and fulfillment also vary greatly from person to person.

Some people find that they're in the mood when they feel really relaxed; others, however, have sex in order to relax and find that they want sex when they feel stressed out, as a way to unwind.

Some find that their thoughts turn to sex when they're already in a good mood, and others use sex to boost their mood.

Some folks desire sex when they're feeling confident and powerful, and others find that they are most in the mood when they feel safe enough to be vulnerable.

It follows that if you're going to become a master of seduction, your approach and skills will need to be adjusted according to the emotions you and your partner(s) associate with sex. If you want to meet their sexual needs, you will need to understand their emotional needs as well—in and out of the bedroom. And, of course, you will want them to do the same for you.

One of the most effective ways to better understand, seduce, and entice your partner(s) involves tapping into their **core erotic feeling**. And if you want to teach your partner(s) how to seduce you, you will want to understand your own core erotic feeling too.

Your core erotic feeling is the feeling you require in order to get in the mood for sex.

SEDUCTION INSTRUCTION

Self-Inquiry: Core Erotic Feeling

Unfortunately we do not have a surefire gimmick or quiz to identify your core erotic feeling (CEF) with precision, but we encourage you to answer these questions to begin contemplating what your CEF might be:

▸ Do you need to feel relaxed in order to have sex?

▸ Do you need to feel loved?

▸ Do you need to feel honored?

▸ Do you need to feel happy and joyful?

▸ Perhaps you need to feel safe, powerful, playful, or stress-free?

▸ Do you find that you are in the mood when you feel sexy and desired?

▸ Do you experience sexual desire when you feel comfortable or when you experience a degree of challenge?

▸ Do you want sex when you are tired or when you are full of energy?

▸ Does sex seem most appealing when you feel vulnerable? Or does it appeal to you most when you feel powerful?

▸ How do you want to feel before you have sex?

▸ What puts you in the mood for sex?

> ▸ How do you want to feel during sex?

> ▸ How do you tend to feel after sex?

> ▸ How do you want to feel after sex?

Think of a recent fantasy. How did you feel? How did others relate to you in the fantasy? How did you relate to them?

Think back to a really hot and memorable sexual experience. What did it entail? What made it so hot? How did you feel during the lead-up to this encounter? How did you feel during and after this experience?

As you explore the emotions associated with past sexual experiences and fantasies, you will likely be able to identify emotional themes. You will probably observe that there is a specific feeling (or two) that you tend to associate with peak erotic experiences. Try to narrow them down to identify the feeling that is *indispensable* to sex for you—the emotion without which sex simply isn't going to happen.

After considering these questions, how do you most naturally fill in the blank?

In order to (possibly) have sex, I need to feel _____.

We've put *possibly* in parentheses as a reminder that experiencing your core erotic feeling does not guarantee that you will want to have sex or that you will proceed to have sex, but simply that you are more likely to be *open* to sex. So if you want to be open to sex, you will want to do the things that help to cultivate your core erotic feeling, and if your partner wants to be open to sex, they will want to cultivate theirs too. Ultimately, it's up to you to access your CEF—your partner plays an important role too, but you need to begin with yourself.

NONEXHAUSTIVE LIST OF CEFS:

Happy. Powerful. Confident. Desirable. Sexy. Loved. Safe. Honored. Relaxed. Stressed. Challenged. Jealous. At-risk. Empowered. Subjugated. Playful. Energized. Serene. Excited. Rested. Calm. Vulnerable. Sexy. Comfortable. Nervous. Daring. Inspired. Passionate. Liberated.

How to Cultivate Your Core Erotic Feeling

Once you have identified your CEF, it is *your* job to make changes and shifts in your lifestyle, communication, and sex life to support this feeling (if you want to).

For example, if your CEF involves feeling *sexy and desirable*, you need to lay the groundwork to allow yourself to feel this way. Consider . . .

What daily activities make you feel sexy/desirable?
What daily activities detract from this feeling?
How do fundamental activities (e.g., sleeping and eating) affect this feeling? Can you make any small adjustments?
When do you feel most sexy/desirable?
Who are the people that support you in feeling sexy/desirable?
What messages do you receive that make you feel sexy/desirable?

What messages do you need to address that detract from feeling sexy/desirable?

When was the last time you felt sexy/desirable? What were the circumstances and how can you recreate them?

How do you hold yourself back from feeling sexy/desirable? What can you change moving forward?

You can also ask your partner for support and show them how to make you feel sexy and desirable. They shouldn't detract from these positive feelings, but it is also not entirely their responsibility to ensure that you experience them. Some people don't like the language of instruction, but we believe that you have to teach your partner how to make you feel sexy (or another feeling that is important to you).

▶ Tell them *what* you want to feel.

▶ Tell them *why* you want to feel it.

▶ Be *specific* about how they can help you to feel this way.

Real Folks Explain Their Understanding of Their Core Erotic Feeling

I just need to feel **relaxed**. I cannot be thinking about work or kids or family or anything else that stresses me out. So what I've learned is that I have to cut myself off from work a few hours before we go to bed. If I keep checking the emails, I'll still have my head in the work game and sex is never going to happen.

Donna, 29

My girlfriends and I have talked about this and so many of us agree that we want to feel **desired**—like the object of desire. If you make me feel sexy, I'll probably want you too. I know you're going to tell me that I have to make myself feel sexy too, and I know you're right, but really the thing that pushes me over the edge enough to actually have sex is when my lover lets me know that they really want me.

Jas, 31

I've always had a strong sex drive, but once I've been with a partner for a few months, I tend to lose interest. I think it has to do with being comfortable and knowing that I can have them. I guess I like the chase and that's why the CEF concept makes sense to me. I need to feel some sort of **challenge** in order to really want sex. If there's no risk, I'm just not feeling it.

Leilani, 30

As a straight guy, I don't really have the same opportunities to feel hot or **desired** (even saying this sounds cheesy, which reminds me of how gendered our expectations are when it comes to sex). My girlfriend gets it everywhere she goes—she'd probably say it's too much (which I totally get), but for me, no one really tells me that they want me. And with all of my exes, our sex life was really reflective of gender stereotypes, so they expected me to come on to them since I'm the guy. It would always get to the point that I'd be frustrated or bored, because I never got the chance to feel desired, and I was always the one dealing with rejection. The framework of the CEF makes things clearer for me: I want to be wanted, and my girlfriend can make me feel wanted just by looking at me, touching me, complimenting me, and flirting. That's how I want to be seduced. I do the same for her, but in a different way, because she wants to feel challenged. It's actually a good fit, but we still switch it up because I know what it's like to always be the seducer, and I don't want her to get bored.

Paolo, 27

I definitely need to feel **relaxed and destressed**—that's key to seducing me. Help me to relax. Help out with some of the tasks around the house. It's not seductive in a sexual way, but it is part of it. When my partner helps with dinner, dishes, or even organizing our finances, I can relax and get in the mood for sex—whether I'm being seduced or doing the seducing.

Toby, 38

If you want to really seduce me, you need to make me feel **taken care of**. I do not want to be tasked with responsibilities or feel pressure to perform in any way. I just want to feel like you're willing to take control of the situation so that I can relinquish my need to be in control. It's not that I want to feel dominated. If I had to sum it up in one word, I guess I want to feel catered to.

Juliana, 40

I want to feel **confident**. That's it. And I know what makes me feel confident and what erodes my confidence. On my end, I need to hang out with certain people like my older sister and avoid others like my younger sister. I also need to practice yoga, because it helps me feel more grounded and connected to my body. On my lover's end, I just need her to show up for me—when she's really present, I feel more worthy.

Maxi, 33

If you want to seduce me, make me feel **important**. Make me a priority and really listen. I don't like talking for the sake of talking, but if she really makes me feel heard, I feel more connected to her. So for me, seduction isn't about how you touch me, but how you interact during the day, at dinner, and in all the interactions leading up to sex.

Aftan, 35

I want **attention**! Make me feel like the center of your world, and I'll be eating out of your hands. Look at me. Touch me. Smell me. Talk to me. Talk about me when I'm not around. If you are attentive, I feel sexy and that puts me in the mood for sex.

Lee, 34

As you contemplate and explore your CEF, consider Brian and Jasmine's story:

Brian and Jasmine enjoy sex and have a good relationship. They are kind, patient, and laugh often. They both express the desire to have more sex, but they both struggle to initiate sex, and they consider themselves in a *seduction rut.*

Brian runs a small company and tends to come home stressed out at the end of the day. He has trouble letting go of work-related stressors, and even though he wants to have sex, he struggles to get in the mood if his workload is heavy. He finds that he has intrusive thoughts, and even though he wants to reach out and touch Jasmine, he is preoccupied with ruminating thoughts about his day or about the next day's tasks. Upon considering the CEF approach to sex and seduction, Brian concludes that what he really needs in order to have sex is to feel *relaxed.*

Jasmine also runs a small company, but she doesn't tend to think about work as much when she's away from her desk. She stops responding to emails by 7 p.m. and thinks about sex often. She wants Brian to want her and really show her that he wants her. She gets a lot of attention from other men and women, but she craves sexual attention from Brian. Jasmine has no difficulty expressing that she's most likely to be in the mood for sex when she feels *desired.*

Both Brian and Jasmine struggle with seduction. Sometimes she gets frustrated with the fact that Brian is so often distracted by work, and he finds it difficult to explain to her how he's feeling.

Brian: It's not that I'm not attracted to her. I am. My head is just always so full.

Jasmine: I just want him to show me that he wants me—even if we're not planning on having sex.

Brian: I want her. Obviously. She's beautiful, sexy . . . she's everything. I just need to learn to relax more.

Jasmine: He doesn't tell me this. I need to hear it. Otherwise, I think his lack of interest is because of me.

As we discuss the CEF, Brian acknowledges that he needs to make some lifestyle changes in order to be more relaxed—not just for sex, but for his own health. He commits to shutting off his phone an hour early for the next two weeks to try to create a new habit. He also starts using a mindfulness app to practice being more in the moment and eliminating intrusive thoughts.

Though initially resistant, Jasmine knows that her core erotic feeling cannot be solely Brian's responsibility and she cannot personalize what she perceives as his "lack of interest." She has to do what it takes to feel desirable and show him how to make her feel desired too. She admits that she feels more desirable when she gets dressed and does her hair, but since she works from home, she's often in flannel pajamas and doesn't bother to brush her hair most mornings. Though Brian doesn't care what she wears, she realizes that *she* feels better when she puts a little effort in. Jasmine also reports that she feels more desirable when she masturbates, but she doesn't do it often because she's waiting for Brian to initiate sex.

Jasmine: There's something about how I feel when I'm done touching myself that makes me feel like I can do anything. I feel sexy and irresistible—and that feels powerful. I feel the same way after sex with Brian.

Over the course of one month, Brian and Jasmine implement these small changes: Brian shuts down earlier and uses the app, and Jasmine sets time aside to masturbate and get dressed even when she's working from home.

They also talk specifically about how they want to be seduced, answering the questions in the Seduction Instruction and One Thing I Love About You worksheet, which you will find at the end of this chapter.

The shift for Brian and Jasmine occurs gradually. Though they immediately grasped the CEF concept, it took time to change their thought patterns and behaviors. It wasn't an overnight breakthrough, but over the course of the month, they both reported being more open to sex and also more comfortable initiating sex and seducing one another.

> Jasmine: What I really learned is that I can feel desirable and be the initiator or seducer. My sexuality has been so tied to being wanted that I never put myself out there. I've never admitted to my own fear of rejection. I think all these years I've been waiting around for him to seduce me because it made me feel sexy, but I can actually feel just as hot if I'm doing the seducing—sometimes. To be honest, I didn't even know how at first, but he's a very tactile person and all it really takes is touch. He guided me to slow down a bit and not fondle him right away, and all the buildup now is so much hotter. I've learned how to touch him all over and I don't just grab and knead at him like I used to. It's about how he feels, but also about how I physically approach him.

Brian: I really like sex, but I'm not one of those sex-crazed guys that wants it all the time. I have to get myself in the mood—whether I'm doing the seducing or being seduced—so the lifestyle shifts were more important to me. I know I'm a little intense and I think I've trained myself to thrive in tension, but I never realized how much it was holding me back in this relationship. I have to make a conscious effort to be relaxed, and I'm getting better at it. Jasmine helps too. She's also turning off her phone earlier, which reminds me to do the same. And she plays loud music in the living room and dining room now, which somehow distracts me from work and helps me settle into "nonwork Brian."

Elevated Erotic Feeling

Once you've explored your core erotic feeling and you've spent some time making the adjustments to support its cultivation, you may find that your core erotic feeling comes naturally to you—either because you've done the work or because you and your partner are in sync.

Alternatively, you might be one of the few who wants to have sex (almost) regardless of your emotional state, like Harry from Barbados:

> I listened to your theory of the CEF and it really helped me to understand my wife. But I honestly do not think I have one. I want sex all the time. It doesn't matter if I'm tired or energetic, happy or sad, relaxed or stressed out. Sex either enhances an already good mood or improves upon a bad

mood instantly. I know it may not always be like this, but
it has been this way for forty years.

If you feel you have mastered your CEF or feel that you do not have a CEF because sex is always on the table (like Harry), you may be ready to explore your elevated erotic feeling.

Your elevated erotic feeling (EEF) is the feeling that takes sex to the next level. It makes it more intense in a specific way—this could be related to physical pleasure, psychological thrill, emotional fulfillment, intimate connection, spiritual experience, or any other benefit you personally derive from sex.

For example, perhaps you need to feel deeply loved in order to consider having sex—this is your CEF. And perhaps you are in a relationship in which this is your norm. You almost always feel deeply loved, so you do not have to specifically work to evoke your CEF in order to have sex. You may find that sex becomes *possible* once you feel deeply loved, but sex becomes more alluring and pleasurably overwhelming when you also experience a sense of challenge. When your partner makes you feel loved, but also makes you work for it, your excitement heightens. When they tease you and suggest that they'll withhold sex, your desire skyrockets. When they threaten to withhold their touch, your body responds with both ache and arousal.

This is your EEF in action, and it makes both the possibility and the experience of sex more exciting. In this example, it is the experience of feeling *challenged*, but your EEF could be entirely different.

You do not have to master your CEF to experience sexual desire, arousal, and pleasure in response to your EEF, but they often go hand in hand.

Unlike your CEF, which may be specific and enduring, you might find that your EEF is more varied. You may have many

EEFs. One day you might respond to a sense of challenge, and another, you might be excited by feelings of jealousy. You might want to feel subjugated on Monday and dominant on Wednesday.

Upon consideration of your EEF, you might be concerned that some of the emotions that turn you on and make sex intensely gratifying are subversive or make you feel uncomfortable. They may not align with your personal and/or political values. For example, you might thrive in independence in real life, but have a strong desire to be submissive when it comes to sex. You might have built a mutually respectful relationship, but be turned on by consensual degradation. This is perfectly normal.

Your sexual desires and the feelings you associate with pleasure need not reflect your real-life ideals. The person you want to be on Saturday mornings at your child's soccer game may be different from the person you want to be on Saturday night behind closed doors. You have the right to play multiple roles, and sex can provide the sense of escape required for you to do so.

SEDUCTION INSTRUCTION

To identify your EEF(s), consider the following questions and prompts:

▸ Try to recall an intensely powerful sexual experience. How did you feel physically before, during, and after the encounter? How did you feel emotionally? Was there a feeling that stood out that you might connect to your pleasure?

▸ Are there any uncomfortable or surprising feelings that you associate with sexual pleasure or arousal? You might want to explore if any of these feelings are also exciting.

▸ Do you ever find yourself in the mood for good sex after intense conversations? Can you recall a few of these conversations and identify how you felt? For example, did you feel tense with your partner, which led to a greater desire for a specific type of sex? Or did you feel turned on by conflict and experience a desire to allow the antagonism to seep into the bedroom?

▸ Are there sexual scenarios, fantasies, or experiences that you find uncomfortable? Sometimes latent desire can hide within or overlap with discomfort, and you might be able to explore these scenarios and feelings in fantasy as opposed to reality. We know, for example, that pain can overlap with pleasure and that physical pain and sexual pleasure often go hand in hand. The hormones (including endorphins) released during experiences of pain are the same hormones that surge during sexual pleasure and that promote bonding between lovers. Pain-related adrenaline and dopamine release can create a natural high that allows you to experience pain in different ways, and spikes in serotonin, melatonin, and epinephrine levels are believed to produce a jolt of pleasure. Similarly, emotions that can be uncomfortable can also produce excitement,

> hypervigilance (sensory and otherwise), and arousal, so it follows that uncomfortable feelings can (for some people) spark erotic feelings and desires.

Our anecdotal observations suggest that it may be common for your CEF to be rooted in comfort and your EEF(s) to be tied to feelings of discomfort. For example, you might identify feeling safe as your CEF, but really find the feeling of risk intensely exciting. You might also find that any variance from your typical relationship roles can be subverted for pleasure via an EEF; perhaps you make all the decisions in your household, so you are really excited to see your partner as a dominant in the bedroom.

This, of course, is not always the case. Feelings of love, safety, and relaxation can also elevate your erotic experience, so you will need to be honest with yourself and communicate your insights to your partner.

LOVERS' INQUIRIES

Now that you understand the roles your emotions play in sexual desire, arousal, pleasure, and fulfillment, you likely have more specific ideas with regard to how you and your partner want to be seduced. But as with all sexual exploration and communication, understanding emotional seduction is not a one-shot deal. Your desires and boundaries will change over time, so you will need to keep the conversations flowing freely and encourage your partner to do the same.

Complete the worksheet and use it to start a conversation with your partner about emotional seduction.

Lovers' Inquiry:
One Thing I Love About You

▶ One thing I love about your body . . .

▶ One thing I love about your voice . . .

▶ One thing I love about your energy/aura . . .

▶ One thing I love about your touch . . .

▶ One thing I love about your personality . . .

▶ One thing I love about your character . . .

▶ One thing I love about how you interact with others . . .

▶ One thing I love about how you treat me . . .

▶ One thing I love about your . . .

Lovers' Inquiry:
Emotional Seduction

Complete this worksheet on your own, and feel free to add to and edit each statement to reflect your interpretations and lived reality. When you are done, feel free to share it and discuss your answers with your lover(s).

When I feel _____, I may want you to seduce me by _____.

When I feel _____, I may want to seduce you by _____.

When I feel _____, I'm probably not open to being seduced. An exception might involve _____.

When I feel _____, I'm more likely to be in the mood for these types of sex: _____.

When I feel _____, my thoughts tend to turn to sex.

When I'm feeling tired, I want you to _____.

When I'm feeling sad, I want you to _____.

You can support me when I'm feeling sad by _____.

When I'm happy, I feel _____ about sex and I want you to _____.

When I'm stressed out, you can help me by _____. I'd prefer that you do not _____.

You will know I'm feeling confident when_____.

You will know I'm feeling insecure when _____.

You can support me when I feel insecure by _____. I'd prefer if you don't _____.

A feeling I struggle with is _____.
When I feel this way, you can support me
by_____. It may not be helpful if
you_____.

HOW TO SEDUCE
WITH CONFIDENCE

Science confirms what almost everyone knows: confidence is sexy. Folks of all genders are drawn to lovers who are comfortable in their skin, but there is no universal path to develop and convey confidence. Some people draw confidence from the company they keep, and others bolster their self-esteem by cultivating skills in the professional and/or personal realms. For some people, confidence is strongly tied to their physical health, while others derive confidence from emotional and cognitive strength. It's up to you to determine how you can be more confident—not just for the relational and sexual benefits, but because you deserve to love yourself!

Confidence, however, is not a permanent state. You can be confident at 8 a.m. and feel insecure by lunch. And that's okay, because confidence can be developed and reinforced via habit. Researchers believe that our brains can be trained to be more confident via synaptic connections. Our brains are comprised of neurons that communicate with one another via synapses, and each time we practice or experience confidence, our synaptic connections may be altered. The theory suggests that when we think confidently, our brains become accustomed to experiencing confidence. When we think positively about ourselves, we engage the circuits involved in pleasure and reward, and it elevates our mood as well as the moods of those around us. They respond to our positivity and confidence, and their response (e.g., kindness, compliments, attention) provides an external source to reinforce confidence. So when we think positively about ourselves, we're training our brain to experience confidence as a habit both internally and via external response sources.

Like all good things, boosting your confidence pays off both in and out of the bedroom. Confidence makes you more likable, positive, influential, and better prepared to manage stress and reduce anxiety. Confident people are also rated as more attractive and successful, but more importantly, confidence is tied to your overall well-being. Research suggests that confidence is positively correlated with higher health measures and longer lives, as it is also tied to happiness and positive emotions (e.g., joy, enthusiasm, gratitude) that support mental and physical health.[7]

If you are ready to invest in your confidence to reap the rewards that extend far beyond the sexual realm, consider some of the strategies below to get started today. You do not have to embrace each approach (they will not all be a perfect fit for your current situation/lifestyle), but try to commit to one that feels manageable and get started right away.

#1. Absorb compliments

Pay attention to the nice things people say about you and repeat them to yourself as soon as you hear them. We tend to focus on negative feedback, but if you keep track of all the positive affirmations and compliments you receive, you will find that they far outnumber the negative.

Some of our clients opt to keep compliment journals or add a section in their regular journal to keep track of compliments.

You can reread these sections at the end of the month or flip through them when you are having a rough day as a reminder of just how great you really are.

SEDUCTION INSTRUCTION

At the end of the day, when you are brushing your teeth, look in the mirror and repeat a compliment you received today or earlier in the week. You may not be mindful of all the compliments you receive (online, at work, in public, at home) and you may even ignore these positive affirmations without realizing it, so make a mental note to pay more attention in the days ahead. And you do not have to wait, because we have one for you now: **You rock. You deserve pleasure, passion, and love!**

#2. Get to know and appreciate your body

The way you feel about your body is tied to general self-worth, sexual self-esteem, sexual functioning, and sexual pleasure. When you are comfortable in your skin, you are more likely to have a fulfilling sex life, as positive body image is linked to positive sexual functioning. If, however, you are unhappy with your body, intrusive negative thoughts can impede sexual response and orgasm. It makes sense that you will be less likely to lose yourself in the bliss of orgasm if you are too busy worrying about stretch marks or criticizing the shape of your tummy.

Oftentimes, we confuse body *image* with body *appearance*, so it's important to remember that *how you feel about your body* is what matters most. It doesn't matter what your body looks like as long as you are comfortable in your skin and feel worthy of love and pleasure. This doesn't mean that you have to idealize every square inch of your body at every moment to embrace positive or neutral body image, but learning to appreciate your body—for its physical, utilitarian, and erotic value—can counteract feelings of unworthiness and lead to greater overall confidence.

To shift the way you see your body, try one new physical act that allows your body to move and perform. You might dance in the dark to your favorite song, or you might allow yourself to get lost in an evening of self-pleasure. Alternatively, you could perform one sun salutation right now and take note of how your muscles feel after just one round. Other options include going for a short walk (get off the bus two stops early or park two blocks away from work) or taking the stairs instead of the elevator to appreciate the fact that you can challenge your body in new ways. Incremental changes to your physical routine can have a significant impact on body image within weeks of implementing the new habit.

You may also want to look at how you can make movement a part of your regular routine via a new exercise regimen. Physical activity isn't only tied to body image in terms of the impact it can have on your overall health and energy levels. More importantly, when you move, your body releases feel-good chemicals that elevate your mood, reduce stress, and can even improve cognitive functioning (e.g., memory). Even short-term exercise can positively affect how you feel about your body, and research suggests that just six workout sessions can lead to feeling healthier and more satisfied with your body (even in the absence of any visual changes to your body).

And finally, if you want to feel better about your body, you might want to consider being more mindful of the images you consume. Your digital diet can positively or adversely affect your body image and self-esteem, depending on the types of content you consume. For example, if you follow and engage with accounts that celebrate diet culture and emphasize that your self-worth should be tied to your size, shape, and weight, it follows that you will (subconsciously or consciously) tie your sense of self to these same attributes. Similarly, if the accounts you follow depict beauty as exclusively thin, white, cisgender, heteronormative, and able-bodied and you do not fit into these narrow prescriptions, you may struggle to admire your own beauty. If, on the other hand, you make a conscious decision to follow accounts and brands that celebrate beauty and sexuality from more diverse perspectives, you will likely find that you come to appreciate and honor bodies of all types—including your own.

You can praise and honor your body in its current state *and* desire to improve or change it based on your own personal standards. This means that you can appreciate your body and still have specific goals that relate to your body. For example, you might appreciate your strength, but want to increase the weight you can bench-press or the number of pull-ups you can master. You might be comfortable with your shape and enjoy the process of working out, and also want to see more definition. And you can be comfortable in your own skin and opt to style your hair or apply makeup to enhance your look.

However you approach positive body image, be kind to yourself and practice compassion—the way you would with a best friend, sibling, or child. You don't have to love everything about your body every single day, but bear in mind that being grateful for and respectful of your body will make you a better lover by helping you to feel better about yourself when it comes to love, sex, seduction, and relationships.

SEDUCTION INSTRUCTION

Go out of your way to adjust your digital diet today. Unfollow accounts that do not inspire you to like yourself as well as those that suggest you need to change your body to conform to an arbitrary cultural standard. Actively seek to follow accounts that celebrate you or inspire you to be your best self.

#3. Surround yourself with positive and confident friends, family, and peers

Much like happiness, science suggests that attitudes toward relationships, sex, and our bodies may be contagious. Research reveals that our own body image and emphasis on weight loss is linked to our perception of how our friends feel about their bodies.[8] So avoid commiserating with friends about weight lost or gained, and hang out with people who do not make their appearance a central focus. Other research suggests that confidence, kindness, and compassion can be contagious too, so make a conscious effort to spend time with folks who are kind to themselves and to others. Confidence may be sexy, but kindness is another key to lasting relationships and sexual attraction.

Research reveals that kindness is linked with higher ratings of physical and facial attractiveness, and a recent study found that those who are more altruistic have more sex and receive more attention.[9] These findings were more pronounced for altruistic men, who also reported a greater number of sexual partners and higher rates of casual sex. You may not associate kindness with sexual attraction and frequency, but it makes sense that what we value in a sexual partner reflects the qualities we seek in a life partner.

SEDUCTION INSTRUCTION

The next time a friend or coworker starts complaining about or criticizing their body, consider speaking up. Most people love compliments, so complimenting them on something you like about them, while acknowledging what they're saying, can be helpful. For instance, if a friend says, "I hate the size of my butt," you could say "I know you hate the size of your butt, but I think it's a great size and I find it to be proportionate to your body." You're not saying that they are wrong, but you are reminding them that there are people who view them as beautiful and you are one of those people. Spark the idea that they are beautiful, and over time, they may embrace it too.

If you're not comfortable speaking up with compliments, you can also change the topic. You are not required to engage in any conversation, and you may want to consider whom you surround yourself with, as your friends' body image affects your own.

And if they often complain about their body (or criticize other people's bodies), you might remind them that you aren't interested in body shaming, because there are so many other interesting topics with which to engage.

Breaking the cycle of negative body talk is subversive but powerful. As you disengage from speaking negatively about your body, you will also begin to *think* less negatively about your body, which creates more openings for viewing your body in a positive light.

#4. Practice gratitude

Gratitude is a powerful feeling that is linked with a host of health, relational, personal, and even professional/financial benefits. When you take notice of the people, experiences, and things for which you are grateful (external sources), it creates a habit of positive affirmations that will apply internally as well. The practice of gratitude is linked with improved health, greater happiness, higher self-esteem, lower rates of anxiety and depression, pain relief, and improved sleep.

You may opt to practice gratitude on your own (e.g., start a gratitude journal) or you may go out of your way to express gratitude in your relationships to address the gratitude gap—you feel thankful but you do not say it. Sometimes you don't express gratitude because saying it might suggest that you *need* help—and make you feel vulnerable. Sometimes you avoid saying *thank you* because you do not feel worthy. Sometimes you avoid expressions of gratitude because you subconsciously worry that you're not reciprocating and do not want to call attention to your own deficits.

But *expressing* appreciation is just as important as *experiencing* it in relationships. And the benefits are layered—they get a boost in self-esteem from receiving the compliment/thanks, and you reap a similar reward in terms of heightened confidence. You also feel more connected to one another when you express gratitude, which may make you more comfortable with sex and seduction.

> **SEDUCTION INSTRUCTION**
>
> Identify something for which you are grateful in your relationship (with a lover or a friend) that you have yet to express in words. Commit to articulating your appreciation via text, email, or in person at the next available opportunity. If you won't see them for a few days (or weeks), put it in your calendar with an alarm so you will not forget.

#5. Masturbate!

Experience breeds confidence, and what better way to gain sexual experience than to have sex with yourself? When you masturbate, you learn about your own body's responses and become more comfortable with the sounds, smells, movements, and reactions that are unique to your body. You also learn to associate these natural responses with pleasure, which can put you at ease when you eventually play with a partner. Moreover, when your body performs for you in any way—whether through exercise, movement, or sexual pleasure—you tend to feel more connected and at ease in your own skin.

The stigma around masturbation, however, continues to exist, so many of us rush through masturbation as a means to an end instead of enjoying the process. Consider slowing down, experimenting with new techniques, and changing positions during solo sex, and you will likely learn to appreciate it as an experience as opposed to a performance. This can elevate sexual confidence by reducing performance pressure—when alone or with sexual partners. (Learn more in the upcoming section on mindful masturbation.)

#6. Accept that you have a lot to learn

We all do!

Nothing holds us back sexually more than the erroneous belief that we are natural-born lovers, as this simply is not the case. Since each person has a unique set of wants, needs, and limitations, which shift and evolve over time, every new lover and encounter presents a fresh course in seduction, affection, and pleasure.

If you sometimes wonder what to do to entice your lover, you are perfectly normal, so do not be discouraged. As sexologists, we have spent years studying sex and we have barely scratched the surface. You're in good company. Accepting that there is no such thing as a sexual mind reader can help to boost your sexual self-esteem and serve as a reminder that the only way to masterfully seduce a partner involves embracing the role of the lifelong learner. If you've made it this far and you are still reading, you are well on your way to continuing to grow and evolve as a masterful lover.

#7. Laugh!

The most confident among us can laugh at ourselves, and when it comes to sex and relationships, a sense of humor may be almost as important as communication itself. This may be why humor is rated as a sought-after trait among all genders. Oftentimes, dating, seduction, and sex do not go as planned, and though they can be serious topics, looking on the lighter side can help relieve the pressure and boost your confidence in bed.

In fact, if you are going to try something new (e.g., seduction that involves role-play), laughter can lower stress levels and give you the confidence boost you need to push through the initial awkwardness. Experts theorize that laughter in humans may have developed as an evolutionary mechanism to assuage anxiety and convey to others that our intentions are harmless.

When it comes to sex, laughter can promote relaxation, which has the potential to improve sexual response (e.g., circulation, erection, and orgasm).

#8. Ask for positive feedback

Sexual communication styles vary, and some lovers will ply you with compliments while others will just lie back and relish silently in the fruits of your labor. If you are not getting the praise you need and deserve, tell your lover(s) to step it up and sing your praises! We all need positive reinforcement—especially when it comes to sex—so make sure you are effusive in your audial response too. One of the best ways to get what you want is to give more of it first.

Consider these lines to encourage them to give you feedback during sex:

> *Do you like this?*
> *How does that feel?*
> *Tell me you like it . . .*
> *Make some noise if you want more.*
> *Tell me how good it feels.*
> *You love it, don't you?*

Also talk to you lover(s) outside the bedroom so that you both understand the mutual benefits of positive feedback.

> *When we're having sex, it feels good when you say . . .*
> *I like to hear the sounds you make, so please don't hold back.*
> *When I hear you groan, it makes me feel . . .*

#9. Turn yourself on first

When you are aroused, your inhibitions and aversion to risk tend to plummet.[10] Arousal not only overrides feelings of disgust, but if your nervousness or lack of confidence is derived from the fear of taking a risk or being rejected, getting turned on can attenuate these feelings.

In one study of 90 university students, researchers found that reluctance to engage in uncomfortable activities is reduced when subjects are sexually aroused.[11] Participants were divided into three groups, and each watched a different film: women-centered erotica, extreme sports, or a generic clip of a train. They were then asked to complete a set of tasks ranging from wiping their hands with a dirty tissue to drinking juice with a bug inside, as well as sexual tasks like lubricating a vibrator. The group who watched the erotic film (the aroused group) was most willing to comply and reported the lowest levels of resistance to the unpleasant tasks.

Obviously, we're not suggesting that sexual seduction is unpleasant, but oftentimes we avoid it because we feel uncomfortable and want to safeguard ourselves against the potential of rejection. One potential way to assuage these concerns involves fantasizing, touching yourself, or using a toy to get yourself aroused *before* you engage in sexual seduction. It may seem counterintuitive to get turned on *before* sex (we often see sex as the means to becoming aroused), but it is not uncommon for arousal to lead to desire, as opposed to desire spawning arousal.

SEDUCTION INSTRUCTION

Confidence-Building Activity

Self-awareness can help you to build confidence around sex and seduction. For example, if you tend to overanalyze things, it's likely that you are aware of this because someone has told you about it (or many people have mentioned it). Recognizing a potential flaw in yourself can help you to identify and capitalize on its upsides. With any habit or trait, there is almost always a balance between its benefits and drawbacks, and we can use this balance to become better partners, lovers, and human beings.

Write Down Your Flaws, Affirmation-Style

Positive affirmations are short statements you say to yourself in the present tense in order to verbalize your hopes and intentions. You can say them out loud or write them down to reinforce them and to increase your belief in their manifestation. Oftentimes, we get caught up in negative self-talk and it becomes our norm. If this is your experience, you may struggle with this exercise, but be mindful of the fact that being uncomfortable is often a positive sign, as growth occurs in discomfort.

I. To begin, write down three things about yourself that you perceive as negative. Write in the present tense beginning with I . . . or I am . . .

For example:

▸ I always worry about the worst-case scenario.

▸ I am always comparing myself to other people.

▸ I am too quiet during sex.

2. Next, identify the positive elements of your negative perceptions.

No personality trait or habit is one-dimensional—therefore it cannot be entirely positive or entirely negative. For example, being extremely friendly may be perceived as positive, but a friendly person may also struggle to set and recognize boundaries, they may reveal too much, or they may expect others to be equally outgoing, resulting in letdown and judgment. Similarly, there are benefits associated with always worrying about the worst-case scenario. For example, you might be better prepared, plan more effectively, and be cognizant of multiple outcomes or consequences; you might also be more mindful and appreciative of the present knowing that things could be worse. Likewise, if you always compare yourself to other people, you may be more likely to learn from them, draw inspiration from their experiences, and operate from a place of humility and respect; you may also learn to appreciate your own circumstances if you compare yourself to those who may not be as fortunate as you. If you believe you are too quiet during sex, you may also notice that the sounds that you do make are authentic and not performative; you may find that you are present and thoroughly enjoying the experience without the need to perform.

Consider your original statements and **identify the upside** of your perceived negative traits to rewrite the affirmations in present tense.

For example:

- ▸ I'm always prepared for anything that could happen.
- ▸ I'm able to observe many different kinds of beauty in the world.
- ▸ I feel present and in my body during sex.

Reconsidering your perceived negatives as positives does not mean that you must embrace every part of yourself or defy opportunities for growth. If you perceive a trait or behavior as negative, in addition to considering the upside, identify ways in which you can change and improve. We are all imperfect and we can always improve.

3. If you would like to change a perceived negative trait, make an effort to recognize and name its opposite, so that you can strive to achieve or embody it.

For example, the opposite of "I always worry about the worst-case scenario," might be "I am hopeful in every experience that I have," or "I trust that everything is fine." It can be helpful to first identify the antonym of the key word in the original (negative) statement (e.g., *hopeful* and/or *trust* replace *worry*).

The opposite of the original statements might read:

▸ I trust that everything is fine.

▸ I accept myself, and I'm happy with who I am.

▸ I love to talk during sex and give great feedback.

As you identify the positives and recognize the opposite of your perceived flaws, make an effort to counter the negatives with multiple positives. Research suggests that in relationships, five positive interactions for every negative interaction create enough positive balance to foster fulfilling connections; apply this five-to-one ratio to your positive-to-negative thoughts as well. Do not stop at one positive affirmation, but pile them on to reap their benefits.

4. Once you have acknowledged your positive affirmations, say them out loud to strengthen your belief in yourself. Repeat your positive affirmations three times in front of the mirror right now.

How do you feel when you say each statement? Really evaluate your feelings to see how your body responds when you say them.

Do they sound believable to you? Why or why not? If they don't sound believable to you, that's perfectly okay. The idea of the exercise is to get your brain trained and on the right track to achieve your confidence goals. Not only are these aspirations, but they are also manifestations, and soon you will see the change that you've wanted all along!

Do you think this could be a part of how you can transform your thoughts? Why or why not? As noted in quantum physics, we can easily change the structure of something based on our thoughts, so the energy that you give to your sexual confidence is sure to help you act and behave in the future according to those transformational thoughts.

We understand that talking to yourself in front of the mirror can feel awkward, but over time, not only will the exercise flow more naturally, but your affirmations will become more believable and real.

Boosting Your Confidence

To further bolster your confidence, write down nine additional positive affirmations in the present tense. These may be qualities or behaviors you currently embody or those you wish to embrace in the future. Read through a few of ours for inspiration:

I am kind and loving.

I am open to learning.

I treat all people with respect and go out of my way to make others feel seen and important.

I smile at strangers and I see that it brightens their day.

I do important work in my community.

I am very funny.

I have made a real and meaningful impact through my work.
I bring positive energy into almost every room.
I take good care of my family.

These nine affirmations, in addition to the six above (the *upsides* and the *opposites*), bring your total affirmations to fifteen; fifteen positive affirmations amounts to five times the original (negative) affirmations you started with just a few minutes ago. This is a great start, as you have achieved your five-to-one positive-to-negative ratio already.

But your work is not done. We want you to continue to add to this list by identifying five positive traits or attributes specifically related to sex (and/or relationships). These positive affirmations may be current beliefs or desired beliefs that you want to manifest. These are a few of our own:

I indulge my lover's fantasies with a very open mind.
I am often open to sex.
I love going down on my lover, and I consider myself skilled and willing to learn.
I feel great about my body; it brings me so much pleasure.
I am almost always willing to try something new.
I initiate sex and make it a priority.

Repeat your own affirmations twice a day. If this seems like too much, record them on your phone and listen to them while you brush your teeth, walk your dog, or travel to work. You might even sing them to a tune in your head (if you are delightfully gifted). Train your brain to hear and believe them. If it feels uncomfortable, it's likely because you are growing.

If you are nervous or uncomfortable with seduction or find yourself in a rut in terms of trying new approaches, it's likely related to your overall and sexual confidence and a fear of rejection. But if you invest in your confidence, you will find that your sense of (sexual) self improves, and you will learn to see rejection as a natural part of life. If you swing and miss once, you have two more strikes before you strike out, and if you strike out, you always have another at-bat. Confidence carries you through to your next opportunity at the plate. Even the professionals do not bat at 100 percent, and the best in league cannot consistently maintain a .500 average, but their confidence ensures that they show up again at the next at-bat, the next game, and the subsequent season.

So go easy on yourself and know that the more you believe in yourself, the better you will be in bed.

SEDUCTION INSTRUCTION

Be your own superhero! One of the best ways to transform your inner confidence involves beginning with your outer self. The way you stand, pose, and move affects how you see yourself and how others perceive you, so strike a superhero-inspired power pose right now and see how it makes you feel in your mind and body. Choose any superhero you admire—from

Superman to Storm—and emulate their body language in front of the mirror. How do you interpret their pose and confidence? Are your hands on your hips? Are your shoulders back? Are you standing straight up with your neck long and your head up? How does being in this position make you feel? Start your day with a fifteen-second pose for one week and see how it affects your self-image and mood throughout the day. Jot a few notes in your journal to track whether or not (and how) this exercise works for you.

SEXUAL SEDUCTION AND VALUES: TWO IMPORTANT LOVERS' INQUIRIES

Now that you have considered seduction from multiple perspectives, it's time to continue the conversation with your partner(s) about your *specific* desires related to seduction. For the two Lovers' Inquiry activities below, set aside fifteen minutes to prepare and make notes on your own, and then carve out additional time for you and your partner(s) to share and discuss your answers with one another.

It is unlikely that you will cover everything in one shot and most people prefer to divide the discussion into multiple conversations. Some of us love talking and asking questions, while some of us may feel like it's an interrogation. Be mindful of your partner's feelings and body language, and move at a pace that works for you both. Conversations related to sex can be emotionally draining, so take breaks and remember that breaking it down into multiple chats can be beneficial in terms of information retention and revisiting topics.

Discussing your desires helps you to improve understanding and respect. You will benefit from sharing both your general and specific expectations to ensure that you're on the same page and to reduce misunderstandings. But it's important to note that even after discussing sex at length, you may still misinterpret your lover's desires, and you can recover from missteps.

One of our clients realized this after an incident involving spitting.

They were in the shower and she was giving a blow job to her boyfriend. It was incredibly raw and passionate and very fun and nasty. He got so into it that he spit into her mouth. It was a total turnoff, and she freaked out, because it wasn't something they had discussed. They worked through it, talked about it, and now they can laugh about it, but they agree that it would have been better to have considered the specifics of their mutual desires in advance.

Unfortunately, most of us do not consider and talk about our specific sexual desires, and instead we cruise along hoping for the best. In doing so, we miss out on sexual opportunities, and this can lead to the belief that we're incompatible, which often builds resentment. This, of course, can be addressed by simply asking questions, sharing insights, and listening to each other from the onset. However, new relationship energy (NRE) often discourages us from having these conversations; we are so caught up in the emotional high (i.e., a surge in dopamine) of meeting a new partner that we make the illogical assumption that sex will automatically work out. Over time, as the dopamine levels stabilize, we realize that no degree of chemistry or attraction can replace honest dialogue.

The good news is that it's never too late to start conversations about sex, so we encourage you to begin now—whether you have been with your lover for two days or twenty-two years.

LOVERS' INQUIRY:
SEDUCTION INTERVIEW

What are the best and worst times to initiate sexual contact?

- ▶ When do you like to have sex? What time of the day is best?

- ▶ Do you like to be woken up for sex when you are asleep?

- ▶ What are the best days/worst days of the week to have sex?

- ▶ Are you open to having sex while you are menstruating?

- ▶ Are you open to having sex while on a work break, or would you rather wait until you're finished with work?

- ▶ What are the best/worst times to have sex as it relates to the kids?

Can you think of a scene from a show or movie that represents the type of seduction you desire? Example: *I like the way Megan told Don Draper of* Mad Men *that he didn't deserve her as she teased him with kinky play. I like the idea of being teased and mysterious at the same time.*

- ▶ Is there a scene that you would like to reenact?

- ▶ Are there shows, movies, or particular celebrities that turn you on?

▸ Have you seen a show or movie in which the romance feels believable?

▸ Are there romantic shows or films that accurately represent your seduction style?

▸ Is there a character you find attractive? What attracts you to them?

Can you think of a scene from a show or movie that represents what you do not want when it comes to seduction and initiating sex? Example: *I hate the aggressive way they kiss on TV with their hands all over each other's faces.*

▸ Are there particular shows or movies that turn you off?

▸ Is there a celebrity that completely turns you off when you watch them on TV or at the movie theater?

▸ Is there a character you find sexually off-putting? Why do they turn you off?

Are there words or phrases you like to hear that might put you in the mood for sex? Example: *I love to hear you declaring your love for me in public.*

▸ If there are words or phrases, what are they?

▸ Should the words be romantic or raunchy? What's the ideal situation for either of these?

▸ Do you like to hear the same words or phrases, or should they be different each time?

▸ Should the words be conversational or can they be one-sided?

What types of touch do you prefer during the seduction/early phase?

▸ Do you like more platonic touches (arms, shoulders) first?

▸ Are you a fan of being in close intimate proximity?

▸ Do you like to begin with light or aggressive touch? Can you describe what this might look like?

▸ Do you like to kiss first to feel it out, or would you rather wait and build up toward a kiss on the lips?

▸ Where do you like to be touched when we first approach each other?

What types of touch should I avoid?

▸ Do you like soft or firm touch? Where do you like to be touched in each way?

▸ Is there a certain amount of pressure that you prefer?

▸ Do you like the feeling of nails against your skin? Where do you like this type of touch?

▸ Do you prefer lots of hair, trimmed hair, or no hair against your skin?

Which areas of your body should I avoid?

▸ Are there any parts of your body that produce or experience physical pain?

▸ Is there a place on your body that you associate with emotional pain?

▸ Are you ticklish, or are there ways of touching that you don't like on certain parts of your body?

How do you need to feel in order to be open to being seduced?

▸ Do you need to be completely relaxed before you can be engaged?

▸ Do you like to be playful or do you like to be more serious?

▸ What feelings do you associate with seduction?

Are there any cues I can look for that might indicate that you're open to being seduced/approached?

▸ Are there any words or code phrases that we can use to hint at being in the mood?

• *Can I use the words ___ to signal my interest?*

▸ What are some cues I can look for when you are in the mood to seduce me?

• *Can I give you some ideas on how you could help me get in the mood?*

▸ Are there any cues I can look for that might indicate that you're not open to being seduced/approached?

LOVERS' INQUIRY OR SEDUCTION INSTRUCTION: SEXUAL VALUES

You can reflect upon these questions in your journal and/or you can share your answers with your partner(s) as part of a Lovers' Inquiry. If you opt to discuss your answers, be mindful that your partner may not be comfortable with some of your answers if they reference experiences with other/past lovers. Similarly, you may be uncomfortable with their responses if they describe pleasurable experiences that don't include you. Consider whether you can explore the experience of *compersion*, which refers to deriving delight from your partner's pleasure—even if it does not include you. If this doesn't appeal to you, let your lover know in advance. You may agree to only share a selection of answers and revisit the ones that give rise to tension or jealousy at another time.

Current Sexual Values:

What I really like about sex is . . .
What I find challenging about sex is . . .
Sex is important to me because . . .
What surprises me about sex is . . .
I would describe my sexual style as . . .
A good sexual connection requires . . .
During sex I usually feel . . .
After sex I usually feel . . .
What I like about my body is . . .
I feel desired when . . .
Lately I feel turned on when . . .

I feel excited about sex when . . .

I feel nervous/hesitant about sex when . . .

One thing I'd like to better understand about sex is . . .

A memorable sexual experience involved . . .

The last time I masturbated, I thought about . . .

In my opinion, this is how sex is different today than when we first met:

The best or most fulfilling sex I have ever had involved . . .

I often think about sex with . . .

CHAPTER

9

EROTICIZING DAILY INTERACTIONS

Many of our clients struggle to make time for sex and seduction in the context of their busy lifestyles. They like sex. They are attracted to their partners. They have happy relationships. But they just cannot seem to make sex happen, and they want to know how to prioritize eroticism when they're busy with work, friends, family, health, and more.

The short answer: recognize that you are not a light switch, and neither is your partner.

The long answer (we hope you have a while): you cannot be turned on and off with the touch of a button, and neither can your partner, so if you want to have hotter, more frequent sex, you need to consider your daily interactions to ensure that seduction and foreplay begin long before you enter the bedroom (or laundry room, or wherever you choose to get it on).

Do you move through life as roommates, coparents, or business partners? Or do you interact as *lovers*? Do you enjoy the moment when your bodies brush together as you pass in the hallway? Do you flirt when the opportunity arises? And do you take the time to look at your partner like a juicy piece of meat—a fine fillet? (Or tofu, if you are a vegetarian?)

You can't go from talking about how you're going to balance your budget or complaining about a nosy neighbor to tearing one another's clothes off with the flip of a switch. And so, an important component of seduction involves setting the scene and weaving eroticism into your daily interactions.

When we suggest that you eroticize daily interactions, we're not suggesting that you make everything sexual. You don't need to make every banana, zucchini, and peach the object of sexual innuendo. *Oh yeah. You eat that banana. You eat it sooo good.* That's not what we have in mind. What we're referring to is ongoing playfulness, fun, levity, and flirtation to ensure that your relationship doesn't dissolve into one of roommates or platonic partners who get less (satisfying) action than the banana itself.

If you want to eroticize your daily interactions, you have to go out of your way to do so. It doesn't just happen. Just like wanting to eat healthy doesn't put healthy food in your mouth, wanting to have a hot sex life doesn't put a penis in your mouth (or a pussy in your mouth, or a boobie in your hand, or a finger in your butt). The best of intentions do not produce results. Actions produce results, and so we present you with a wide range of action items you can use to make your day-to-day dealings more erotic and lay the groundwork for sexual seduction.

Cut Back on Complaining

We know. The weather sucks, traffic is ridiculous, and your coworker's nattering is driving you up the wall. This all may be true, but your partner doesn't need to hear about every single frustration you face on a daily basis. Complaining is neither interesting nor attractive, and it is the antithesis of foreplay. You wouldn't show up to your first, second, or fifth date complaining about your day or bemoaning the humidity, because you wouldn't want to leave a negative impression on a potential partner—and your current partner deserves the same courtesy.

This doesn't mean that you shouldn't speak up when something serious is bothering you or that you need to pretend that all is right in the world. Complaining can be good for you because negative feelings like frustration and disappointment serve a purpose: they help you to identify what you value, what you want, and what you might want to change. When you complain, you acknowledge the emotion you are experiencing, and you need to acknowledge it in order to start reconciling it. Complaining can feel cathartic, and studies suggest that when you accept defeat or crisis, you are better off a year later than those who pretend to be positive.

However, you don't want complaining to drive your conversations or become the basis for connecting in your relationship. And sweating the small stuff (weather, traffic, a rude server or barista) can snowball into venting for hours every day. The more you complain, the more you become accustomed to complaining—from a neurological and habit-based perspective.

To limit your complaining, consider using the *complaint dump*. This is an exercise that allows you to share your frustrations and get your complaints off your chest at a specific time. We suggest you set aside five minutes when you get home to vent about your day's frustrations. You might need five minutes each or five minutes total, and as you become more mindful of your complaining, you will likely find that you will need less time. You will likely learn to address the issues that matter and let the little things go.

Try to whittle your complaints down to two minutes at the end of the workday and then call each other out if you slip into complaint mode later in the evening or on the weekend. As you shift the conversation away from the unnecessary focus on perceived negatives, you will create space for eroticism, playfulness, and flirtation.

Upgrade Your Greetings and Goodbyes

How do you greet your partner? When they walk through the door, do you make eye contact, smile, and take a moment to enjoy being physically present? When you say goodbye, do you take a moment to kiss or embrace as you would if they were leaving on a flight? The little interactions matter, and your greetings and goodbyes set the tone for how you will interact later in the day or week.

Think about how a dog greets you (or its owner). The dog waits longingly for you to walk in. They gaze from a distance and rush to be close to you. They wag their tail, open their mouth, and push their body as close to yours as possible. Can you be more like a dog? Can you take sixty seconds to convey love and enthusiasm for your partner as they depart and return each day? A long hug or kiss can shift the energy in your relationship for the entire day. Research suggests that twenty seconds of hugging[12] or thirty seconds of eye contact can result in an oxytocin boost, which is associated with enhanced feelings of safety, trust, love, and connection—all of which increase the likelihood and quality of sex.

Getting bawdy with your lover(s) as you pass by them in your home is a great way to intimately connect. Sometimes, it's the little displays of affection that enhance your greetings and goodbyes and help you to emphasize your shared erotic energy.

Text Playfully

Rather than texting to update them on your day or ask them to pick up milk, send playful drip texts and riddles. For example, you might send them incomplete messages starting in the morning—

one line from a song you love at 9 a.m. and then an image that reflects your mood at 10 a.m., just to keep them guessing.

Alternatively, you can create riddles to showcase your thoughtful and playful side. Hide a new pair of underwear or a small gift under the front seat of their car and text them riddles that they have to decipher to find their prize.

Sext Them Photos of Other People—with Consent

Look for erotic photos or videos that turn you on and send them incomplete images, GIFs, or short clips throughout the day. Be sure that these photos and videos are consensually in the public domain. Of course you can send pics of yourself (you are hot!), but changing things up adds the element of unpredictability that is likely to pique their interest and start new conversations. If you do opt to send photos of yourself, ensure that you are of legal age, as there are legal consequences for sharing photos of anyone who is underage (even yourself).

Leave Love and Sex Notes in Unexpected Places

It is easy to get caught up in the day-to-day of work and personal responsibilities, so much so that you start acting like roommates instead of lovers. One way to remind yourself and your partner of your intimate connection involves writing down your sexual feelings and desires and sharing them at unexpected times. You can send them via text, email, social media, postal service, or even use your finger to leave a short note on a steamy mirror while they're in the shower.

SEDUCTION INSTRUCTION

Take five pieces of paper and write five messages to your lover to affirm your love, attraction, and connection. Hide them in various spots in your home (or their home), car, bags, or other locations you can access (e.g., their office). You might place them in a drawer they only access once in a while, the bottom of their purse or briefcase, the glove compartment of their car, the back of their armoire, the linen closet, the laundry room, the pantry, or the pocket of an off-season coat. The hope is that they will find them at random intervals and be reminded of the connection you share.

You can make the content of your notes as sweet or sexy as you would like. Here are some examples from our friends and clients:

- Wherever I am today, know that I'm thinking of you—lovingly and naughtily.

- I want to lick you from head to toe.

- I'll be thinking of your soft lips today and every day.

- When you come home, I'm going to bend you over and take care of you just how you like it.

- You are too hot. I cannot get you out of my head.

- I cannot get enough of you—in every way!

- You are the most beautiful creature I've ever laid eyes on, and I love that I get a piece of you for myself.

- ▸ I want to get naked with you—and a few of our friends. ;)

- ▸ I'm yours for the night. Tell me what you want.

- ▸ Tonight, I want you to undress and wait for me in the bedroom.

- ▸ I think of you when I wake up every morning and before I go to bed every night.

- ▸ You are mine. I adore how naughty you are.

- ▸ I love sucking you. I cannot wait to have you tonight.

- ▸ (In a lunchbox) This is only part of your lunch. Meet me at my office at 1p.m. so you can eat the rest.

- ▸ I love the way you sound when we make love.

- ▸ It drives me wild when you adore me.

Reset with Two Minutes of Physical Intimacy

Life sometimes spirals out of control, and we forget to take the time to connect—emotionally and physically. This two-minute activity can help you to feel more present in your own body and more connected to your lover's.

Sit or lie next to one another with your foreheads touching and start to breathe in sync for eleven deep breaths. You may feel uncomfortable and distracted at first, but as you slip into the third and fourth breath, you will likely start to feel more relaxed and close to one another.

Research shows that when you touch your lover, you experience a physiological "interpersonal synchronization" as your heart and breath rates align and pain subsides. Skin conductance, a common method of tracking physical and emotional arousal, also syncs when you sit close to your partner.

So go ahead and get in sync. And if it takes longer than eleven breaths to sync up, do not fret. Stress from the day, distractions, work, your mood, your general health—all of these factors affect connection, so don't put pressure on yourselves to experience a specific result right away. Simply commit to engaging in the process and see how you feel. You may feel the tension subside and be reminded of how close you felt in the past, or you may feel frustrated with the activity altogether, and that is okay. You can try it again tomorrow if today is not your day. The fact that you're willing to try it (again) demonstrates that you are committed to working on your relationship and suggests that you will see improvements over time.

Have Intimate Conversations

You likely speak to your lover every single day, but do you really engage in intimate conversations that create space for vulnerability and spark passion? Do you talk about your jobs, schedules, and families, or do you discuss your deepest fears, personal dreams, and most profound hopes? Oftentimes, the death of passion in relationships occurs when conversations become reduced to mundane reports and updates. *This is what I did today. This is what I'm going to do tomorrow.*

Obviously, many of these conversations are required from a logistics perspective, but they do nothing to spark passion, fuel eroticism, or ignite a sexual connection.

Intimate and vulnerable conversations, on the other hand, can lay the groundwork for an erotic connection, as they help you to see your lover as multidimensional; they're not just the person who forgets to hang up their towel or shows up late to meet you, they're also someone who dreams of visiting Mecca, gets nervous watching golf, laughs out loud while watching movies on a plane, and has a weakness for hamster videos. New revelations and reminders may not specifically turn you on, but they make your partner more interesting and (potentially) appealing. Novelty and the unknown are tied to feelings of passion and desire, so consider engaging in conversations that help you to uncover new discoveries about your partner's past, present, and prospective future.

LOVERS' INQUIRIES

Set aside a few minutes to explore the questions in these two Lovers' Inquiries. Take turns asking each question so that you alternate who asks and answers first, and feel free to allow the discussion to flow freely. If you prefer, you can commit to one question per week over the course of the next few months or use these questions to spark discussion on your next car ride, plane trip, or date night.

Lovers' Inquiry: Provoking Passion

▸ Whom do you admire most and why?

▸ What global issues concern/consume you?

▸ What did you daydream about as a child? What do you daydream about now?

▸ When was the last time you felt really excited?

▸ What is your fondest memory?

▸ If you could change one thing about your teenage years, what would it be?

▸ When do you feel most loved?

▸ If you had one wish, what would it be? (You cannot ask for more wishes.)

▸ If you never had to work, how would you spend your ideal day?

▸ How would you describe an ideal day in the context of your current life?

▸ What is your first memory of when we met?

▸ If you could have a drink with anyone in the world, whom would you choose and why?

▸ When you retire, how do you want to spend your days?

▸ Name two things you love to do that don't cost much/any money.

Lovers' Inquiry:
Initiating Intimacy & Vulnerability

▸ What is your greatest fear?

▸ What do you believe about death and the after-life (if anything)?

▸ What was the highlight of your childhood?

▸ What was your greatest struggle as a teen? How have you overcome and grown based on this experience?

▸ When do you feel most confident? When do you feel most insecure?

▸ Would you change anything about your upbringing?

▸ What do you regret most?

▸ What issue(s) do you struggle with that might surprise people who don't know you?

▸ What can I do to make you feel more loved?

▸ Close your eyes and picture your happy place. Describe it to me.

▸ When do you feel closest to me? Be specific.

▸ How can I show you that I appreciate you?

Take Your Compliments to the Next Level

One-dimensional compliments (e.g., *You look nice today*) might help you charm your way to a better table at your local hot spot, but when it comes to sex, you're going to want to step up your game. Weave **compliments of pleasantry** (e.g., *You are so sweet*) throughout your daily interactions and throw in a few **flirtatious compliments** (e.g., *Wow. You must have been turning heads all day in that dress!*) to show appreciation for sex appeal. Finally, seal the deal with some **animalistic compliments** (e.g., *I cannot resist the perfect curve of your hips. You drive me wild!*) that let them know that you want *them*—not just sex.

Prioritize and Plan for Sex

While spontaneous sex might arise with ease when you first get together, planning ahead is almost always required in long-term relationships if you are both busy with work and personal commitments. Research suggests that foreplay and seduction should begin twenty-four hours in advance of sex, so that the amygdala, the part of the brain associated with processing emotions, is prepared to set worries and stress aside in favor of pleasure and arousal.

The involvement of the amygdala in sexual arousal helps to explain why many of us cannot transition seamlessly from mundane interactions to erotic engagement—our bodies and our brains need to be primed for sexual activity in advance. So if you want to seduce your lover in the evening, start at breakfast with affection (e.g., a passionate kiss), expressions of admiration (e.g., *I love staring at you*), and sexual flirtation (e.g., a gentle brush against the thigh). And do not forget to set the scene. You will be surprised how far a few candles or a romantic soundtrack can go. Which brings us to our next suggestion.

Create an Erotic Lair

Sex and real estate have a great deal in common in that it all comes down to location, location, location. In fact, where you opt to seduce your lover and where you have sex can be just as important as how you do it. Most of us have limited real estate and cannot afford a red room or sex chamber in our humble abodes, but we can tweak the lighting, furniture, and props to ensure that our bedrooms are conducive to erotic pleasure.

Play with color to enhance the mood. Red decor and lighting is believed to excite the senses, while whites and blues are believed to be calming. Switching your light switch to a dimmer is one of the most affordable and simple ways to set the mood, and strategically positioned mirrors will appeal not only to visual lovers, but to those who like to get kinky with positions and props. You may not be ready to invest in a sex swing yet, but try to purchase extra pillows that can be used to prop up your bodies into more varied positions. If you find the pillows help you to get more creative, consider purchasing a wedge pillow like the Liberator wedge/ramp combo, which provides lift for multiple angles and lots of soft padding for comfort all around.

And keep those phones, tablets, and computers out of the bedroom if possible . . .

Create Spaces That Are Work- and Tech-Free

Technology can enhance erotic interactions if you are using apps to flirt (check out In the Mood to set a date with your mate) or texting as a form of foreplay. But when devices distract you from being in the moment, research confirms that the costs to the quality of the relationship are significant,[13] so be mindful and purposeful about how you consume digital content when you are with your partner(s).

Whether you opt to ban your devices from the dinner table or ensure that your bedroom is free from electronic devices, you are likely to reap the benefits in a matter of days. Research continues to confirm that digital technology detracts from presence and connection even when you are not actively scrolling or typing. The mere presence of a phone detracts from concentration, presence, connection, empathy, and trust.[14] This may be because phones serve as a distraction and create the urge to check in, seek additional information, and draw yourself away from the present moment. One study found that when phones are on the table or in our hands, one-on-one conversations become less fulfilling, and empathy declines.

Additionally, the light emitted by phones, laptops, and tablet devices is considered "short-wavelength enriched," which means that it can interfere with the sleep-support hormone, melatonin. The costs of poor sleep include a greater likelihood of conflict the next day, poorer conflict resolution skills, and decreased interest in sex.

Snuggle (Naked)

Cuddling and other forms of physical affection are important in most relationships, because physical affection is one of the ways we express love, desire, and commitment. In North America, for example, we tend to reserve most forms of physical touch for those we love, and many of us are touch deprived. One study found that those who lack affection (and crave more physical affection) experience lower levels of happiness and higher levels of loneliness, depression, relationship dissatisfaction, and stress.

Some of the benefits of cuddling include the release of feel-good hormones (e.g., oxytocin) to boost your mood and a decrease in cortisol, which is associated with stress. One study found that the benefits of cuddling are not fleeting, and that they mirror those of sex; those who engage in sex or physical affection experience less stress and a happier mood the following day,[15] and those who receive more hugs from a partner have lower blood pressure.

Couples who are more physically affectionate report higher levels of love, fondness, and relationship satisfaction,[16] and when you express physical affection, your partner is more likely to see you as likable, trustworthy, and composed. Research also suggests that cuddling can help stave off and improve the management of conflict.[17]

While snuggles can heighten intimacy and erotic connection, it is important to note that if you only cuddle as a means to a specific sexual end, you may find yourself feeling unfulfilled, as research suggests that cuddling only leads to sex 17 percent of the time.[18] However, physical affection for the sake of the experience itself can strengthen the relationship overall.

For most of us, it's important to engage in both sexual and nonsexual affection, because at some point, you may stop having sex temporarily (e.g., during busy work periods, after childbirth, or when grieving); if the only time you are affectionate is during (or prior to) sex, you may stop being affectionate altogether. This is a common experience for couples who have trained themselves to reserve affection and cuddling exclusively for sex play. Cuddling, of course, is only one form of affection, but it is a particularly beneficial one.

If you want more cuddles and your partner isn't much of a snuggler, talk to them about your desires. Make a request without complaining. This is the mistake most of us make: we wait until we're frustrated to express (or identify) our own needs, and then we complain, as opposed to making constructive requests. When our partner recognizes a complaint, they are more likely to ignore it, withdraw, or become defensive instead of listening and responding with support. Consider adapting the following language to reflect your needs and style:

I love when you hold me from behind. It reminds me just how strong you are.

When you hold me, I feel closer to you. It really helps me to destress.

I'm so stressed out. But when you touch me or kiss me, it helps me relax.

Kiss my forehead. It makes me feel loved.

Let's cuddle. It's my escape from the pressure of the real world.

We used to lie in bed all day. And it almost always led to sex. I want more of that. Can you block off Sunday for lazing around?

SEDUCTION INSTRUCTION

Oftentimes a lack of physical affection results from busy schedules or a lack of understanding of our partner's (and our own) desires. To address or curtail potential misunderstandings, talk to your partner about what you want using the following prompts to guide you:

▶ On a scale of one to ten, how important is physical touch to you?

▶ How does your family express affection? How has this shaped your desire for touch?

▶ How do you like to be touched? For example, do you want to cuddle naked or simply hold hands while we watch a movie?

▶ Are there times when you crave more touch? Are there times when you prefer not to be touched?

▶ Do you want me to touch you more often? Show me how.

These are practical questions, and you can adapt and add others as they arise. Just as you ask dinner guests about their dietary restrictions and preferences, so too should you ask intimate partners about their preferences when it comes to affection, cuddling, and other expressions of love.

Note on physical touch: You have a right to ask for what you want, but your partner is not obliged to meet every one of your needs. In fact, **no single person can**

be expected to fulfill every one of your needs, from the emotional and practical to the social and sexual. You ultimately have to take responsibility for yourself and seek out multiple sources of support. For example, if you want more physical affection and your partner wants less, you may consider how your friends, pets, kids, and professionals (e.g., massage therapists) can also contribute to your desire for physical touch.

Touch Your Partner When You Are Not in the Mood

One of the most meaningful times to be physically affectionate is when you don't want to be. This doesn't mean that you should do anything against your will, but if you can break through the frustration, anger, exhaustion, and resentment and just reach out and touch one another, you will likely find that reconnecting physically will help you to reconnect emotionally; these negative feelings that interfere with an erotic connection may subside as your body responds to the power of touch.

Stare at Their Best Assets

It's okay to objectify your partner within the context of a loving, respectful relationship. You can honor your partner *and* love their breasts. You can respect their intellect *and* lust after their booty. True love and animalistic lust need not be mutually exclusive.

In the early stages of a relationship, physical admiration and desire for your partner are fueled by curiosity, nervousness, and the desire to uncover the unknown. You lust after your new love interest as you subconsciously fill in the ambiguities to idealize your potential mate. Over time, however, the primal desire evolves and real life takes over. We stop *looking* at our partner as a lover and begin to regard them more as a person who plays multiple roles—best friend, roommate, confidante, coparent. And though it is absolutely desirable to see your lover as a complete person and not just a sex object, maintaining a piece of animalistic admiration for them will sustain the erotic connection over the long term.

The next time your partner walks through the door, do not ask about their day or talk about your schedules. Instead, stare at their best assets. Soak in the sex appeal that first attracted you to them. Stop what you're doing, focus on what you see in the moment, and *look* at your lover. Pick a body part you love and focus on it like an animal in heat.

Try this when they annoy you too. Did they leave a tiny drop of milk in the jug and put it back in the fridge? Instead of muttering under your breath, think about their biceps. Is their laundry strewn across the bedroom floor? Pick it up for them as you visualize their soft breasts.

Forget about all of their annoying habits and *objectify* them. Lay on the compliments and be flirtatious. Make a conscious effort to shelve whatever conflict, tension, and stress exist for a few minutes at the end of every workday and just admire them for their physical assets. This will not always lead to sex, but it will remind you that underneath those tiresome habits lies a body that excites you and brings you pleasure.

Avoid Dialogue That Is Self-Pitying

Complaining to identify needs is one thing, but self-pity and self-deprecation wreak havoc on sexual interactions. When you start conversations with self-pity, it can be antiseductive. Self-pitying phrases include, "I haven't had sex in a while, so I don't remember how to do this," "I'm really not good at this," or "I feel like an amateur compared to you." These statements signal to a potential lover that the sexual experience probably won't be good, and they may lose focus; rather than enjoying the experience, they will likely feel pressured to respond to and counter your self-pity.

Revisit Your Early Relationship

Why Do I Love You Again? involves a trip down memory lane. It is a simple way to revisit and reignite the attraction you experienced when you first met.

Set aside thirty minutes with your lover and ensure that you eliminate all potential distractions. I know it's tough, but this is a partnered exercise and isn't intended for the wide world of social media, so shut down your devices and take some time to slow down. I didn't believe it myself until I tried it, but somehow the Twitter-verse manages to survive without us while we take time to recharge.

You can complete this exercise one of two ways: take turns answering the following questions face-to-face or, if you prefer, print them out and jot down your responses before sharing them.

LOVERS' INQUIRY:
WHY DO I LOVE YOU AGAIN?

Take some time to reflect and try to be as honest as possible as you respond to the following questions. Feel free to share your answers with your partner.

▸ What was the first thing you noticed about your lover?

▸ What first attracted you to your lover?

▸ On your first date, what excited you most?

> ▸ On your first date, what made you nervous?

> ▸ Do you remember the first time you kissed? What was it like?

> ▸ Do you remember the first time you had sex? What was it like?

> ▸ What is one awkward intimate moment you wouldn't want to relive but are able to laugh about now?

> ▸ Can you remember the wildest/hottest sex you ever had? What made it so memorable?

> ▸ How has your partner changed for the better since you first met?

> Other options for recalling the feelings and sexual tension of your early days together involve retelling the story of how you met, reenacting your first date, visiting the location of your first kiss (or other memorable first), listening to your song under the covers, or simply talking about hot sexual memories from your past.

Do Not Complain About Your Body

This is a life changer. In a world that profits from teaching you to dislike your body, liking your body is a revolutionary act. When you complain about your body, it can detract from your partner's appreciation and admiration of it. For example, if you complain about your butt or tummy, they may assume that you want them to avoid touching these areas. And when you complain about your body, you both become less present and mindful. For instance, if you complain about your body in bed, it can divert their focus away from the experience at hand as they try to reassure you or respond to your complaints.

When you like your body, your partner is likely to be more at ease with their physical appearance, as body image is contagious.

The next time you catch yourself ready to complain about your body, try one of these five approaches instead:

1. Think about what you like about your body. Do you appreciate your skin, your hair, your toes, or the shape of your calves? Identify one thing you like (or think about a feature you know your lover likes) and repeat it to yourself. *I love the way my skin feels. I love the way my butt looks in jeans. I like the way my skin glows after sex.*

2. Pay attention to the function and performance of your body. Does it support you in the realm of dance, fitness, hiking, sex, or another physical activity you enjoy? Does it take you places or allow you to connect with people in physical spaces? In your mind (or aloud or on paper), show your body gratitude by thanking it for a specific performance, function, or activity. *Thank you for allowing me to sway to the beat of the drums. Thank you for allowing me to move at will. Thank you for carrying me to far-off lands. Thank you for allowing me to volunteer in my community.* Your body is the vessel that carries you through life, and learning to appreciate it for its function as opposed to its form may help you to feel more connected to and grateful for it.

3. Use the ninety-nine rule. Consider whether or not your current concern about your body will matter when you are ninety-nine years old—especially within the context of your relationship. Will you be worried about your stretch marks or forehead lines when you are lying in bed after nearly a hundred years on the planet? Or will you be grateful for the time you spent with your loved ones? Will you wish you had spent more energy worrying about the shape or size of your body, or will you be grateful that it served you for so many years?

The ninety-nine rule can also be helpful when you are facing conflict and tension with your partner. Consider the issue and contemplate whether or not it will matter to you when you're older. Will you remember why you were fighting or what point you were trying to prove? Some issues are worth addressing, and will improve when you engage in conflict. Others, however, are trivial and will not matter in the long run. The ninety-nine rule can help you to keep things in perspective.

4. Talk to yourself as you would to your best friend, a sibling, or a child. You wouldn't bash your best friend's body or disparage your own in front of a young child. Show yourself the same respect you show others.

5. Compliment someone else. When body bashing is on the tip of your tongue, try redirecting your focus to someone else— your partner, a friend, a coworker, or anyone else in your presence. When you give a compliment, you improve social interactions and make them more enjoyable, elicit reciprocal warmth and positive intentions from others, and get a boost in self-esteem and positive emotions.

Just as performing acts of kindness can reduce anxiety, alleviate pain, and even lower blood pressure, giving genuine compliments can reduce negative feelings (and beliefs) as you redirect your focus to something positive.

Play Pranks
Be playful and bring levity to your daily interactions whenever possible. Laughter can set the mood for erotic interactions, and couples who are more playful have more exciting and fulfilling

sex. Playfulness comes in many forms. You might simply joke around at the breakfast table, sing silly songs in the car, wrestle them into bed, or play lighthearted pranks (e.g., changing their ringtone to your best karaoke version of "I Want Your Sex").

Another option involves playing the Sixty-Second Spit challenge. One partner fills their mouth with water and tries not to spit it out while the other partner does everything they possibly can to make them laugh for one minute.

However you play, let it serve as a reminder that life and sex do not always have to be serious.

Use a Role Ritual to Shift into Your Lover Role

We all play a variety of roles in our relationships and day-to-day lives. Oftentimes our professional, social, and familial roles come to define us, and our roles as lovers tend to take a back seat. Using a role ritual at the end of the day or before you begin your weekend (or time off) can remind you both that in addition to being friends, roommates, community members, coparents, and partners, you are also lovers, and you deserve to indulge in this role without guilt or distraction. A role ritual signals a shift from your public role(s) to the private, more sensual one you play exclusively with your partner(s).

Your role ritual might be most effective if it helps you to relax, enjoy yourself, and be the best version of yourself. You might pick a song, mix a cocktail, change your clothes, switch your phone off, write in a journal, close the blinds, stretch, read a few pages of a book, adjust the lighting, or shake it out on your living room dance floor—it's entirely up to you. Whatever ritual you choose, allow it to serve as a reminder that you no longer need to think or talk about work, kids, chores, or your schedule; instead, relax and enjoy quality time with yourself and your partner. Performing the role ritual doesn't mean you have to have sex, but simply that you commit to spending time together as lovers—touching, smiling, laughing, and connecting in an intimate way—however you define it.

Share Daydreams

Just as talking about sexual fantasies can enhance connection, understanding, and the erotic charge in your relationship, so too can allowing your minds to wander into nonsexual fantasy territory. Do you dream of winning the lottery and imagine exactly how you would allocate the funds? Do you reminisce about your younger years as an athlete and daydream about what life might have been like had you gone pro? Perhaps your mind wanders to a fantastical world in which you live among the animals, at one with nature? Whatever you dream about during your waking hours, consider sharing some of your most untamed thoughts with your lover(s) and indulge in the dopamine high associated with anticipatory and/or hopeful daydreams.

By offering your lover(s) a glimpse into your most personal reveries—however luxuriant or impractical they may be—you will likely broaden their understanding of the way you think and the feelings you yearn to fulfill. Your daydreams may reveal a side of you they have yet to see, and the novelty of the revelations can reignite passion and desire as they see you in a whole new light. This can improve daily interactions outside the bedroom and has the potential to lead to new conversations related to both personal and sexual fulfillment.

Admire (and Even Flirt With) Others Together

A wandering eye is not the same as a wandering heart, but since monogamy is touted as the ideal and default setting in romantic relationships, you may have been conditioned to desire a lover who only has eyes for you. This expectation of exclusive sexual attraction is not only unrealistic but can lead to disappointment and letdown when you're reminded that you are not the only attractive person on the planet (or on their radar).

The reality is that regardless of the intensity of love or attraction between you, your lover will most likely admire and experience attraction to other people. This doesn't mean that they will want or need to act upon this attraction, but if you both give yourselves permission to be honest about your desires, it can enhance and eroticize your relationship. Many people report that talking about forbidden or taboo thoughts serves to reduce the power of those thoughts and decrease the likelihood of acting upon them.

Experiencing and expressing attraction and admiration for other folks is normal and healthy—even if it makes you uncomfortable. Many couples find that opening up about their natural feelings not only enlivens their attraction to one another, but also deepens connection, owing to the honesty and vulnerability that underpins the associated discussions. You don't have to share every thought or sexual desire with your partner, but consider beginning with a discussion of celebrities you admire or sharing some of the details from your sex dreams (which, of course, are beyond your control).

It's also worth noting that the act of trying to suppress a thought (e.g., a fantasy about someone other than your partner) only results in a higher frequency of its occurrence. The reoccurrence of the thought is called the rebound effect. You may have heard of the white bear experiments. Study participants were divided into two groups: the first group was told *not* to think of a white bear for five minutes and then told they could think of anything they wanted, including white bears, for the next five-minute interval. The next group was simply told they could think of anything, including white bears, for five minutes. The first group—the group that was told to suppress the thought—found that they thought about white bears more often.

If you are uncomfortable with your partner's attraction to other people, acknowledge your feelings and ask yourself why you feel the way you do. What values or messages contribute to your feelings of jealousy, insecurity, or possessiveness? You may be able to ask your partner to offer you reassurance or even make small adjustments to their behavior (if they feel so inclined), but ultimately, you are responsible for managing your own reactions. Remember that jealousy is both a universal emotion and, in some cases, a functional one, as it can help you to identify what you value or aspire to. In most cases, it's your reaction to feelings of jealousy that determines the outcome; the next time you feel jealous, consider using jealousy constructively (e.g., to examine and talk about your feelings) as opposed to lashing out, making accusations, or withdrawing from open communication. And if you're dealing with a jealous partner, lead with empathy, knowing that jealousy is a feeling—not a character flaw.

Play Music in Your Bedroom

Music can move you, and research suggests that those who listen to loud music have more sex![19] Music can shift your mood, improve your perspective, boost confidence, and help you relax—all of which have the potential to heighten your erotic connection. The contagion hypothesis suggests that we mimic what we hear in our environment, so create a playlist that helps to cultivate the emotions you need to feel in order to get in the mood.

Do you want to feel powerful? Listen to heavy bass. Looking to feel amorous? Pick tunes from your early days of dating. Do you need help decompressing at the end of a stressful day? Choose a mellow melody. Is happiness your core erotic feeling? Play an anthem that lifts you up. Identify the emotion that underpins your core erotic script and find the music to match!

SEDUCTION INSTRUCTION

Find your favorite music application and make a love song playlist that you and your lover(s) will appreciate. If you have a smart-speaking personal assistant, you can call on it to play the list any time you want to set the mood!

Schedule Appreciation Check-Ins

Whether you are in a long-term relationship or not, an appreciation check-in is one way to keep you bonded over time. Do this at least once a week to remind yourselves what you love and adore about one another. As a weekly activity, it can help you to reflect more specifically on something they did that you liked or appreciated. We all love to be appreciated, and what better way to absorb that information than while spending quality time together?

SEDUCTION INSTRUCTION

Reflect upon these questions or use them as writing prompts in your journal.

Considering your day today . . .

What kinds of erotic daily interactions did you have?
Did you get to flirt?
Did you send a sexy text?
Were there any missed opportunities with a potential lover?

> *How would you change the day to include more erotic daily interactions?*
> *What will you do tomorrow?*
>
> Remember, it's important both to plan for eroticism and to think on your feet.

However you inject eroticism into your daily routines, remember that sex doesn't just happen—you have to make it happen. If you wait until you're in the mood for sex, the mood may never strike, so make small adjustments to your morning, midday, and evening routines that make you feel sexier and more open to sex. You do not have to do it all. Simply pick one item from this long list of options and get started right now. Don't delay. There's no time like the present.

10

PHYSICAL SEDUCTION
AND FOREPLAY

When most of us think of sex, we think of the physical part first, but sexual pleasure can be drawn from a multiplicity of sources and experiences. We've already discussed a variety of approaches, including the verbal, emotional, and visual, so now it is time to move on to the physical components of sexual seduction and foreplay.

Physical touch is essential to human growth and survival. Some of the potential benefits associated with affection include lower blood pressure, an increase in oxytocin, a reduction in stress hormones, pain alleviation, heightened immunity, and lower levels of anxiety.

Physical touch activates various regions of the brain associated with thought and emotion. Touch is associated with decreased heart rate and blood pressure and with increased oxytocin levels. And the benefits of physical touch flow in both directions—to the giver and receiver. A study found that when women touch their partners as a sign of support, there is more activity in their own ventral striatum, a region associated with reward processing.[20]

As you experiment with physical components of seduction, you don't need to think about why it affects you, but rather *how* it affects you and your lover(s). Different types of touch may be suited to different lovers, different areas of the body, and also different moments in time. The way a partner wants to be touched on Monday night after a long day might be different than how they want to be touched on a lazy Sunday morning. Below, we begin with an exploration of erogenous zones and then discuss a variety of touch techniques you can try on your own or with a partner.

The Hottest Erogenous Zones

Erogenous zones are areas of the body that are associated with sexual excitement and arousal. Of course, the whole body represents one big potential erogenous zone, but there are specific spots that tend to be more sensitive to physical seduction and touch. They vary from person to person, as no two bodies are alike. While you may love a gentle tickle against the back of your knees, your best friend might find it irritating or uncomfortable. This, of course, brings us back to the necessity of talking to the person(s) with whom you are having sex.

We've said it before and we'll say it again: if you want to have *the sex*, you have to talk about *the sex*.

When it comes to erogenous zones, you might find that your most sensitive spots vary from day to day and that your mood, health, partner, and even positioning play a role in which areas are most responsive to erotic touch. For example, Jenni, who identifies as kinky, has a special and tenuous relationship with the nape of her neck:

I can have an orgasm from having my neck and back touched, kissed, stroked, and flogged. But at the same time, I will curl up and recoil if you kiss it at the wrong time or in the wrong way. Sometimes it's actually about the partner and not about me.

So I would say the nape of my neck is both an erogenous zone and a no-go zone, which makes my body a little complicated. This is why before every scene—regardless of whether it's a regular partner or someone new—I have to be very clear about what I'm in the mood for. And during the scene, I give specific directions. Now. Not now. Lower. Higher. I'm very specific. I'll even say I want you to increase the intensity by 10 percent. It doesn't sound sexy when I say it now, but it is hot in the moment, because not only am I in control, but I'm utilizing a part of my body in a way that most people know nothing about. Can you imagine having an orgasm simply from an ice cube rubbing against your neck? It's powerful stuff, but it really does require that I communicate excessively, which is worth it to me.

With the right touch (or touch avoidance), any area of the body can ache with desire and swell with arousal. Consider seducing your partner with gentle, but purposeful touch of the following potential erogenous zones:

Suprasternal notch: This area, located at the center of the neck just above the collarbone, is highly sensitive to gentle touch, and you will not want to apply much pressure, as it overlies the airway. You can pique your partner's interest by simply tracing your fingertips around this notch with featherlight touch. Alternatively, kiss their collarbone with your lips and tongue and then breathe gentle, warm air over this indentation to arouse their interest. The more you prime an area for pleasure, the more likely they'll be to experience pleasurable sensations in the region during heightened arousal and orgasm.

The sides of the chest: The stretch of skin beneath the under-arms can be highly responsive to pressure, temperature, texture, and other forms of touch. Use the backs of your hands to trace your fingernails from under their arms to their hips, or play with a leather or feather prop to heighten awareness of this area while you're working your way down and warming them up for oral.

Philtrum: The entire face can be highly sensitive to erotic touch, and if you've ever experienced an orgasm during which your face tingles, you likely consider your lips, cheeks, chin, forehead, and eyelids highly erogenous. The word *philtrum* is derived from the Latin for *love potion*, and it refers to the sensitive groove right at the center above the upper lip. Try gently brushing up against it with the tip of your nose while you snuggle, or running your lips sensually along it while you kiss.

Belly button: The belly button is not only associated with sexuality for its close proximity to the genitals, but it has a history of primal and erotic associations. It is the giver of life and is rich in nerve endings. It has been painted as both visually and tactilely erotic, and its exposure has been banned as indecent in dress codes as a testament to its taboo sexual associations.

If you play around the edges or stimulate the shallow part of its groove, you may experience pleasurable sensations in the surrounding region across the fibers that lead to your spinal cord, which also relay information from your bladder and urethra to your brain. This is why some folks report feeling tingly sensations in their genitals via stimulation of the belly button and others find that orgasmic sensations are intensified via direct contact with the belly button.

Treasure trail: The path between the navel and the pubic mound can be particularly responsive to erotic touch, and you might find that your hair-grooming practices affect how you interpret these sensations. If your partner has pubic hair, trace your fingertips gently around, swirling to create a bit of heat and friction. If they are bare, use the backs of your fingers to gently awaken their nerve endings, and breathe warm air along the trail with a wide-open mouth to arouse interest and draw awareness to the pelvic region.

Perineum: This is the space between the scrotum and the anus or between the lower vulva and the anus, depending on your anatomy. You might also hear it referred to as the *taint*, *gooch*, or *chode*.

If you have a penis, you may be able to access the inner bulb of its base through the perineum—press firmly with several fingers or a toy right behind the balls. Pulse or slide with pressure or use a vibrating toy.

The We-Vibe Verge is a penis ring that wraps around the base of the penis and balls and vibrates against the perineum. It can be worn in multiple positions depending on your preference, but if you want to stimulate the sensitive penile bulb, allow the vibrating extension arm to press firmly against your perineum.

If you have a vulva, a smooth flat toy like the We-Vibe Touch or a powerful vibrator like the Hitachi Magic Wand can create rumbly sensations against this erogenous area.

Pucker: You do not have to go inside to have anal sex. Good stuff happens on the outside too. The pucker (bum hole) tends to be sensitive to light touch from a finger, tongue, or vibrator. Twirl your way around it before pressing gently on the outside with your thumb, or use your tongue to lick petals around it as though it is the center of a daisy.

Shoulders: Though stimulation of your shoulders is unlikely to result in a deluge of orgasmic pleasure, the shoulders may hold the key to desire and arousal. Many of us harbor tension in this region, so a shoulder rub may be all we need to let go of our stress and feel more connected to both our own body and our partner's.

The nape of the neck and ears: A cross-cultural study of nearly 800 participants found that people of all genders rate the nape of the neck and ears as highly erotic, with a high "ability to facilitate sexual arousal."[21] Plant soft kisses here when you're out in public to build anticipation and give them a taste of what's to come.

Nipples: Folks of all genders can derive exceptional pleasure from nipple play, and some people can reach orgasm from nipple stimulation alone. The genital sensory cortex, which is also activated through stimulation of the vagina and clitoris, may be involved in this process. Research suggests that nipple play releases oxytocin, which induces both relaxation and pleasure. Consider these nonsequential techniques for chest, breast, and nipple play:

▶ Tease by breathing warm air around the area until they are begging for you to suck them into your warm, supple lips.

▶ Slide your lips over their nipple and twirl your tongue all around the areola with a wide, flat tongue.

▶ Curl your tongue around the underside of the chest while you run the backs of your hands down the sides with the softest touch.

▶ Tell them how much you love them! *They're perfect. I can't get enough of them.*

▶ Work your way from the outer edges of their chest, slowly circling toward the center with your tongue, lips, or your favorite sensual prop. You can use your hands, your mouth, your nose, or anything that will create a unique sensation.

▶ Roll their nipples as lightly as possible between your thumb and index or middle finger.

▶ Nibble on their nipples as they approach orgasm, as the pain thresholds can double at this point in the sexual response cycle. The overlap between pleasure and pain can intensify orgasm, and researchers believe that this may be related to the activation of various brain regions including the anterior cingulate gyrus, lateral prefrontal cortex, insula, amygdala, and cerebellum (just to name a few).[22]

▶ Pinch and release their nipples every half second right before orgasm.

▶ Play with ice cubes or Popsicles and be sure to lick up every last drop.

Create your own erogenous zone: Create erotic or orgasmic associations by stimulating any part of your lover's body right before or during orgasm. For example, if you make a habit of stroking the center of their palm while they orgasm over and over again, they may come to associate the stroking of this area with orgasmic pleasure. This learned association connecting an area of the body to peak erotic experiences can come in handy when you're looking to seduce them in the car, at the dinner table, or in bed—a simple stroke of their inner palm (or any other area you choose) might arouse a subconscious interest in sex and/ or signal to them that sex is on your mind.

Not so erogenous: feet. Despite the fact that the foot is a popular fetish and we tend to derive pleasure from having our feet rubbed, research suggests that the feet are not particularly erogenous. In fact, a study published in the journal *Cortex* reveals that the foot ties with the lowly kneecap in terms of its capacity for pleasure and arousal.[23]

Avoiding Your Erogenous Zones

Oftentimes sex is framed as a goal-oriented act with orgasm as the grand finale. It follows that your focus oftentimes narrows to emphasize genital pleasure with the goal of getting off. But what if you were to avoid your hottest spots for a few minutes (or longer)? Chances are, the anticipation and excitement would build into a powerful crescendo of pleasure, and you would naturally find yourself more mindful of the present moment.

The next time you engage in sex play, make your hottest spots off-limits for the first three to five minutes, and then increase the deprivation time as you play with the power of anticipation as a tool for more mindful sex. As you will recall, sexual gratification can be just as intense during the anticipation stage thanks to a spike in dopamine—the neurotransmitter associated with pleasure and reward.

Now that we have discussed some of the most common erogenous zones, let us explore specific techniques to build anticipation, desire, arousal, and pleasure.

Erotic Touch Techniques

As you experiment with new and varied erotic touch techniques, we suggest that you keep a few things in mind:

▶ Carve out the time, space, and energy to try each of these out with your lover(s). When you are in a rush, it can be difficult to really *feel* a new experience, so set dedicated time aside and do not feel you need to test them all in one shot.

▶ Be open to the new sensations and accept that not every approach will work for you. If you don't like a specific type of touch, that's okay. Bear in mind, however, that your body is constantly changing, so what may not work today could turn out to be irresistibly appealing in a few weeks. This constant evolution of sexual experiences is what keeps sex fresh and exciting, so while you should not force yourself to like something, you may want to try it at least twice before you submit your final verdict.

▶ Try them all. Oftentimes, when we suggest a specific technique, we are met with an "are you kidding me?" response. This is because instructions in print and even visual demonstrations cannot possibly convey the physical sensation of a technique. Once you give them a try, however, you might be surprised by the feelings themselves as well as the corollary learning.

▶ Make them your own. Change them. Rename them. Add a twist. There is no right way to perform any technique, so don't get hung up on following our directions to a T. These are guidelines intended to spark *your* creativity.

▶ Check your body. Remember, it's more seductive when you are being hygienic with clean hands, nails, and other body parts that you are going to be sharing with yourself or with a lover. Be sure to check for any scratches and cover up any open wounds that may be involved in your sexual experience.

As you read through, you might try some of them on your arm or thigh for a few moments, or you can read with a partner and pause to take a few minutes with each technique.

The Butterfly Kiss

Warm up your fingertips and slather them in your favorite oil, balm, or massage lotion. Gently flutter them over your partner's skin, alternating between fingers one or two at a time. Consider beginning with their hips and working your way slowly down to their outer ankles. Then work your way back up their inner legs until you reach their inner thighs.

Slow-Motion Pitter-Patter

Similar to the Butterfly Kiss—use the *backs* of your fingertips to create a tingly sensation as you tenderly flutter them along the spine, around the lower back, across the shoulder blades, or down the sides of their chest. Move very slowly and change the pattern and order of how you flutter your fingers every thirty seconds.

The Breath Kiss

The *Kama Sutra* promotes the Breath Kiss as a sensual approach to arouse the interest of a woman and prime her for sexual pleasure; our experience, however, tells us that the same principles can be applied regardless of gender. Breath kisses have the potential to create pleasure that extends across the entire surface of the skin and beyond. The Breath Kiss involves bringing your wet lips as close to their skin as possible and breathing a gentle kiss without touching. Breathe a few warm kisses over the back of their neck at breakfast or dinner. Take them by the hand while you're in the car and breathe sensuous kisses over their inner wrists. While you are warming them up, lick around their thighs and hips to create a wet spot, and then breathe gentle kisses over the moistened area.

The Breath Kiss is among our favorite physical seduction techniques, as these kisses can be planted all over the body and can help eager, well-intended lovers to s-l-o-w down in the heat of the moment.

Remember that you are not blowing out a candle or blowing on dice for good luck; the Breath Kiss involves a gentle but purposeful exhale. You can breathe kisses over the entire body from head to toe. Take your time. Covering every square inch. Because when you stimulate the entire body—even with your breath—you are more likely to create full-body anticipation and pleasure when the time for sex and orgasm arises.

The Reverse Trace

This is an important touch technique for people who tend to move too quickly or too aggressively. Consider setting a timer on this one so that you take at least a few minutes to caress and explore your partner's skin only with the backs of your hands— no grabbing or kneading allowed. Trace your fingers and the tops of your hands across the body slowly, starting at the neck and working your way down. Or start at the waist and work your way up and back to the middle. Vary your touch pattern from straight lines to curved esses to figure eights to more organic movements that reflect your mood. Enjoy the sensation against your skin and take note of how your hands feel when you leave your palms out of the touch equation.

Tantalizing Pulls

Begin with the tips of all five fingers resting gently on the surface of the skin. You can utilize this touch technique across the entire body—from the calves and thighs to the shoulders and small of the back. Little by little, draw all five fingers together toward a center point as slowly as you possibly can, maintaining the lightest touch possible. When you arrive at the center, gradually extend your fingers back out and repeat, inching your way along their skin. You can play with Tantalizing Pulls on their shoulders or scalp at the dinner table, or tease and please around their butt cheeks or breasts as you lie naked in bed.

Effleurage

Use the palms of your hands to massage the entire surface of their body in wide, sweeping circular (or oval-shaped) movements. You can opt to move both hands in unison or alternate between your right and left, keeping both palms pressed warmly against their skin the entire time.

Figure Eights

As an alternative to circular strokes, glide the palms of your hands in sweeping figure-eight patterns across the body. Do not avoid their hot spots, but do not spend any extra time on them as you cover the full surface of their skin over and over again.

Finger Drawing

Draw your physical touch and energy across their body to create heat, desire, and circulation. Cover your hands in your favorite massage oil or lotion and run all ten fingers in a straight line from their neck all the way down to their toes and back up again. Start slowly and gently and gradually increase the speed and pressure. Feel the contours of their body with your fingertips, and consider blindfolding them to help them relax and really sink into the sensations.

The Body Slide

Cover your body in oil or lotion and slide it all along your lover's body. You can have your lover lie on their stomach and slide along their backside or rub your thighs along the length of their legs. There is no one way to master the Body Slide, but in massage parlors, they often slide their body up the full length of the backside before turning their partner over onto their back and sliding masterfully down the front.

Trickle

Use your fingertips to awaken the nerve endings that are most sensitive to light touch: the tactile corpuscles. These mechanoreceptors are primed for heightened pleasure (they do not interpret pain), and you can use the tips of your fingers or the tip of your nose in a circular pattern to spread pleasure along your partner's inner arms, outer chest, or treasure trail region.

Spread Stripe

Start with all ten fingers in the center of their back, stomach, or thighs. Spread them in opposite directions, starting with firm pressure and releasing as you reach the edges, then pull them back together, increasing the pressure as you return to your starting point. Repeat and feel free to swirl your fingers in various patterns as you draw outward and ease up and then pull them back together with firmer touch.

The Wet Trace

Use your tongue or even a finger with lube or massage oil to paint a wet line, and then breathe gently over the Wet Trace you've created. Use an open mouth for warm air, or purse your lips to create a cooler sensation. Temperature play can be highly erotic as you shift between breathing warm air against the skin with a wide-open mouth and cool air with tightly pursed lips to activate your lover's sensitive thermoreceptors.

Grounding

Grounding techniques are used to facilitate presence, and we use physical grounding to cultivate presence through awareness of touch sensations. One simple grounding technique involves connecting through purposeful, firm touch. This can be particularly useful when exploring gentle touch techniques that are unpredictable. For example, if you are gently fluttering your fingers over your lover's chest, pressing your other hand firmly against their thigh or holding their hand can help them to focus on your physical connection and feel more in the moment. If you're working your tongue gently around their abdomen or breathing gentle kisses against their skin, you might consider wrapping your hand around their vulva or thigh to encourage physical connection and grounding.

Two-Handed Heart

Using your palms, slide in an upward sensual motion and then stroke outward to trace the shape of a heart all the way back down to the starting point. You can do this on the back, around the butt, or even over their thighs or calves—in almost any position.

Change of Pace

Warm them up with a firm palm rubbing in a slow, circular motion for six to eight strokes to create a sense of grounding and connection. Then follow up with gentle figure eights with two light fingers over the same area for six to eight strokes to create anticipation and heighten sensitivity. Switch back and forth between the warm, comforting palm and the gentle, less predictable touch for the two-finger figure-eight pattern. Alternate at different intervals—you can switch after three or four strokes, or extend to a dozen strokes per touch pattern to keep them guessing and help draw your focus to the pressure, temperature, rhythm, and movement of your touch.

Hard-Soft Stroke

Using massage oil, pull and press firmly with your knuckles in one direction, and then switch up to a soft, gentle, barely there palm in the other direction. Try this stroke across the body, extending your touch to every square inch over the course of ten to fifteen minutes. When you alternate between various touch techniques and pressures, it can help them to be more mindful and present as they focus on the different physical sensations.

Freestyle

Close your eyes, breathe deeply, and simply touch for your own pleasure. Feel their skin beneath your fingers—pay attention to the texture, the temperature, the curves, and the consistency as you run your hands over their entire body. If space and flexibility allows, bring other body parts into the mix—touch them with the sides of your cheeks, your nose, your chin, your chest, or whatever other body part thrills you. Allow yourself to explore for exploration's sake. Touch for pleasure's sake with no goal in mind. If you take just five minutes to freestyle touch, you will likely find that the way you feel about your lover changes, and the way you see their body shifts as you explore with your eyes closed. You may also notice that the way you feel connected to your own body changes as you focus in on the physical sensations of touch alone and release worries, goals, and expectations.

Kissing

If there is one complaint we hear from folks in long-term relationships—including those who are thrilled with their sex lives—it is that their partner doesn't kiss them enough. I also hear concerns that the kissing simply isn't as passionate, deep, or sensual as it was in the beginning. And this is to be expected.

When you first meet a new partner, you tend to kiss and make out with fervor. You are fascinated by the novelty of the situation and excited by the potential of where kissing might lead.

But over time, as you get to know one another, the allure of making out can subside. It's not that kissing doesn't feel good, but once you have engaged in other types of sex, you may no longer experience the thrill of the unknown that you derived from kissing early on. There are, of course, exceptions, but in the early stages of a relationship, kissing often serves as a prelude to sex, whereas in long-term relationships, it is often a tool of affection. It obviously doesn't need to be this way, so if you want more kissing in your life, speak up and ask for it. Better yet, lean in and plant a kiss on your lover's lips instead of waiting for them to seduce you.

If your partner is not as keen on kissing as you are, consider these approaches:

▶ Make a habit of kissing them right before they orgasm so they learn to associate kisses with peak erotic experiences. Over time, as the erotic association builds, they will likely find themselves more drawn to kissing when they are in the mood for both sex and intimacy.

▶ Compliment them on their kissing skills. Let them know that you are powerfully turned on by kissing, and they'll be more likely to be generous with their kisses. Think back to a kissing experience that you enjoyed and let them know that you are craving more of it. One of the hottest ways to seduce your partner involves asking for what you want—and compliments go a long way. Research suggests that many of us are more motivated by compliments than by rewards of cash, so apply these findings in your relationship to increase your partner's motivation to please.

▶ Experiment with some of the sensual kissing techniques

below to inject novelty into your routine, whether you have been together twenty days or twenty years.

Speaking of getting more of what you want sexually . . . remember to ask for what you want using **compliments** as opposed to **complaints**. "I love the way you kiss me. It makes me weak in the knees. I'd love to be kissed like that when I walk in the door after work," is likely to produce a more positive result than "You never kiss me anymore."

Kissing Techniques

Supersoft Kiss

Gently press your lips together and hold still with featherlight pressure for a few breaths. Slow your exhalations as you breathe through your nose and allow yourself to feel the texture and temperature of their skin against yours. Take note of their breath as you slide their lower lip in between your lips, gliding from side to side as slowly as you possibly can. Take your time and kiss with relaxed lips for a minute or two, allowing your tongues to rest against one another as your breath rate continues to slow.

Lip Trace

Blindfold your lover or ask them to close their eyes. Use all ten fingers to slide slowly and sensually over their cheeks. Hover your lips above theirs for a moment, barely making contact. Trace your tongue around the outline of their lips more slowly than what might come naturally at first. As you relax and your body's natural functions (e.g., heart rate, breath rate, blood pressure) decelerate, the slow trace around their lips' curves will feel more natural. Leave your lips hovered over theirs when you've traced the entire outline, and sensually slide your tongue from side to side between their lips.

Tongue Roll

Tilt your heads to opposite sides and press your lips firmly together. Have them keep their tongue still while you roll your tongue around theirs. Feel the inside of their cheeks and play with their tongue as you kiss, suck, and slurp with passion.

Premium Shelf

Begin by blindfolding or covering their eyes. Take a few minutes to caress their scalp using your fingertips. Even if you're tempted to dive into kissing or reach underneath their clothes, s-l-o-w down. Once you are both feeling relaxed, plant gentle kisses on their ears, cheeks, and neck. Work your way gradually toward their lips and slide their upper lip between your lips. Kiss and suck very gently, working your tongue inside millimeter by millimeter. Slide your tongue back and forth over the roof of their mouth (on the inside) to create tingly sensations in their lips and beyond.

Sweet Spot

Run your tongue along the inside of their lips to glide against the fragile notch of tissue that connects the lips to the gums. This sensitive spot (called the frenulum of the lips) exists on both the upper and lower lip in the center. You are probably familiar with the frenulum of the penis, which connects the foreskin, and you will also find a frenulum attached to the clitoris and at the bottom of the labia.

Old-School Lover

Warm up your hands and place them on your lover's cheeks; have them do the same to you. Kiss with tongue and be mindful of the feeling of their skin against the palms of your hands. Feel its texture, shape, temperature, contours, and movements. The face is highly sensual but often viewed as utilitarian, so consider touching your partner's cheeks as you pass them in the kitchen, when they come home after work, when you kiss good-night, and when they are going down on you.

Undulating Kissing

Kiss gently and slowly with a soft tongue and soft lips for ten seconds, and then increase the pressure and speed for ten seconds. Pull back and undulate between gentle, sensual kisses and more animalistic, deeper kisses; allow your breath and sounds to match your energy, breathing more slowly and deeply while you kiss softly and increasing your breath rate and allowing your sounds to emanate with greater volume as the kissing intensity rises.

Giver and Taker

Take turns being a giver and receiver for ten minutes. As the giver, you will take ten minutes to touch, caress, lick, kiss, and use your breath to stimulate your lover's neck, ears, face, lips, and mouth. Move slowly and touch purposefully. Take your time and cover every square inch of this region. Allow your lips, tongue, cheeks, fingertips, and palms to really *feel* their skin. Enjoy every curve and angle. Notice the temperature changes. Indulge in the textures.

If you are the receiver, sit or lie back in a comfortable position and simply enjoy your partner's touch and energy. Pay attention to the pleasurable sensations and give yourself permission to *take* pleasure as much as you give it. Being a taker in bed makes you a better lover, as you allow your partner to hone and treasure their own skills, luxuriate in your pleasure, and experience their own pleasure derived from your body's unique reactions.

In-Sync Kissing

Press your foreheads together gently, tilting your heads forward so your noses are not squished. Take a few deep, exaggerated breaths, allowing your breath to fall in sync with your lovers'. Move your lips closer together and suck their lips in between yours as you continue to match their breath.

Full-Court Press

Kiss with passion as you press your entire bodies against one another. Allow yourself to really feel the full-body contact, paying attention to the pressure, textures, temperature, and movement of your bodies.

Calming Kiss

Kissing can create a natural high as dopamine spikes, and some people report feeling euphoric after a heavy make-out session. If you want to prolong this high, kiss more slowly and mindfully. Close your eyes and slide your tongue inside, and rather than twisting and twirling, hold it almost still as you breathe deeply. Take note of everything you are feeling. What do you feel against your tongue? How do your lips feel? What are you feeling on the inside of your cheeks? Can you feel their breath with your eyes closed? You may find that your breath synchronizes with your partner's and slows significantly as you both relax and allow yourselves to be in the moment without giving a thought to what's to come.

Code Kisses

Pick a code word or experience, and stop whatever you're doing when you encounter it to give your partner a kiss. If you are on a road trip, you might pick a road sign that leads to a kiss (e.g., signs depicting animals) or opt to kiss at every red light. If you are at an event or party, you might choose a word (e.g., "baby"), and each time someone says it, you find your lover and give them a kiss. Most of us need a reminder to be affectionate, and this type of playfulness may put you in the mood to be seductive or be seduced later in the day.

The Tasty Kiss

One of the most sensitive spots of the lips is the upper lip right underneath the philtrum. With your lover, trade off kissing each other on the upper lip. Not only can this be a playful game of who can get the most kisses in on the upper lip, but you can also add a guttural moan, similar to how you'd moan when you've enjoyed a tasty food choice. These sounds tend to bring a smile to most people's faces, so please your lover with this tasty kiss.

Kinky Kiss

If you are of the kink variety or you want to spice up your sex life by introducing some kink into your life, this is a great way to invoke some energy and passion. When you're with your partner, place your less dominant hand on their cheek, with your palm on their jawbone. With your dominant hand, give them a nice little slap on their other cheek with your fingers and then hold their face as you force your mouth on their lovely lips.

11

THE ULTIMATE PHYSICAL SEDUCTION: FULL-BODY ORGASM PREP

Most of us experience orgasmic sensations in our genital region, and some of us report feeling sensitivity in our bums or breasts. This may be because these regions are hotbeds of sexual activity (and engorge with blood during arousal), but it is also possible that these areas are perceived as orgasmic because they receive physical touch during seduction and sex. But what if you were to extend your touch to other areas of the body? What if you were to pay as much attention to the small of the back, the nape of the neck, and the inner ankles? Chances are you would start to feel a tingle in those regions as well . . .

There are multiple pathways to full-body orgasms, and you may be familiar with the role that the G-spot plays in full-body pleasure. Many folks report that G-spot orgasms feel different than other orgasms (e.g., clitoral orgasms), as the pleasure spreads throughout the body as opposed to being felt solely or most intensely in the genitals. Researchers believe that this may be explained by the fact that the G-spot communicates with the brain via the vagus nerve, which wanders throughout the body. The prostate (P-spot) is reported to play a similar role, and those who enjoy prostate massage report comparable experiences of orgasmic pleasure spreading across their body.

Aside from stimulating the G-spot and P-spot (which we address in the upcoming chapters with a range of techniques), you may also be able to produce intense full-body orgasms simply by touching the entire body—to awaken the nerve endings, promote circulation, and draw awareness to every square inch of the body's sensitive surface. As you touch and draw appreciation to the toes, ankles, knees, thighs, back, collarbone, cheeks, ears, and more during sexual seduction and foreplay, you can increase the likelihood of experiencing orgasmic sensations in these regions when the big ohh finally arrives.

The exploration of the entire body with your hands, toys, props, and lips requires time, so it may not fit into your regular Tuesday evening routine. However, if you set some time aside to entice and delight the entire body through head-to-toe and toe-to-head touch, the payoff can be extraordinary.

There is no perfect formula for touching the body from head to toe, but you might want to start with the scalp and work your way down. We've included some broad instructions as well as a link to a free audio guide below.

Before getting started, choose a space that feels warm, safe, and comfortable. Take a quick scan of the room to clear it of distractions. Remove all electronic devices and pets. If you choose to play music in the background, make sure it is at a reasonable volume and consider instrumental sounds so that you aren't distracted by the lyrics. Set the lighting and temperature to your liking so that you will be comfortable.

Begin by lying next to your partner, holding hands, or sitting in their lap so that you become physically connected. You can kiss, snuggle, or take a few deep breaths as you begin to relax. If you want to experiment with boosting oxytocin, gaze into one another's eyes for two minutes, allowing your facial muscles to soften as you get past the giggles.

When you are both ready, have your lover lie on their stomach in whatever state of undress makes them most comfortable. You can drape a sheet over their body or they can lie naked in front of you.

Begin at their scalp by touching very gently. Roll your fingertips through their hair or trace them in slow semicircles. Kiss gently with your lips and use your nose to follow the contours of their ears. Take your time here, spending a few minutes on their scalp and ears alone.

Work your way down their neck, breathing breath kisses over it for a few minutes; you can keep your hands on their head to stay grounded. Follow the shape of their neck with the tip of your nose, cheeks, and lips. Plant a few gentle kisses and trace around with your palms. Smile as you touch them for pleasure. Use massage lotion or oil and make sure it is open and accessible in case you need to reach for more during the full-body caress.

Work your way down to their shoulders—kiss, lick, breathe, swirl, touch, and really *feel* their skin against yours. Notice how their skin feels and how your body responds as you touch and explore. Use the backs of your hands over their shoulders as you gradually work your way over their upper back and shoulder blades.

Touch with your fingers, palms, lips, tongue, and breath. Be slow and gentle, as you are just getting started. Explore this area by experimenting with different strokes. Try the Slow Motion Pitter-Patter over their shoulder blades and then follow up with the Two-Handed Heart for a few minutes. Pay attention to your breath. Is it slowing down? Can you hear their breath deepening?

As you work your way down their sides and lower back, touch slowly and with intention. Can you breathe warm air all around the small of their back? Can you kiss, caress, and roll your tongue around and then breathe over the wet path? Can you roll your tongue in a figure-eight pattern? When you press your cheeks against their lower back, can you feel their body rise and fall with each breath? Spend a few minutes here before you slide down to their buttocks.

Sweep your palms gently over their cheeks. Allow your hands to move in unison or alternate one at a time. Start slow and gentle, and increase the speed and pressure over the course of three to four minutes. Breathe over their butt cheeks. Kiss them. Suck them. Breathe them in. Slide your finger between them. Glide your nose between them. Roll your tongue around the area. Tease down low, but do not reach around and grab their hottest spots yet. Tickle, trickle, caress, knead, and handle to your heart's content. You are touching to escalate their pleasure as well as you own, so do what feels good for you.

As you work your way down their thighs, alternate between gentle trickles and warm touch, as you wrap your hands right around them and slide up and down. Move from side to side as well as in unpredictable, organic patterns with your lips, cheeks, nose, hands, and chest. Slip your fingers between their thighs so that you almost touch their genitals. Open their thighs and kiss all around with heavy breath. Be sure to explore every square inch so no area goes untouched.

Take your time as you explore their calves, inner ankles, and feet. If they do not like to have a specific area touched (e.g., feet or knees), be mindful of their preferences. You can make exceptions to the every-square-inch-rule to ensure their emotional and physical comfort. Once you have caressed the entire back side from head to toe, move back up their legs for a second round and move on to their arms. Play with the thin skin of their inner elbows and take extra time with their fingers to touch, caress, kiss, and suck. Experiencing orgasmic sensations in your hands can be overwhelming, so spend a few extra minutes here.

Check in with them and with yourself throughout the process. If you find that your mind wanders, or if you have trouble staying present at any time, bring your focus back to your breath and pay attention to the way the air feels flowing into your nose and out of your mouth. After a few breaths, bring your attention to your fingertips, and feel free to close your eyes to heighten the way in which you interpret and experience physical sensations.

When it is time to roll them over, cover their eyes and reconnect by holding hands or kissing before starting again from head to toe. Spend at least a few minutes caressing their face with the backs of your hands. Plant kisses and breathe deeply. Kiss and caress their neck, ears, and collarbone.

Work your way down their body just as slowly as you did on the back side, exploring and experimenting with new touch patterns. Follow the curves of their chest, abdomen, and hips. Roll your fingers around the nipples, breathe over their chest, kiss down their sides, slide your cheeks under their arms, trace their contours with your nose, use a feather or soft scarf over their shoulders and upper arms, turn on a vibrator on the bedside table to pique their interest, swirl your palms over their inner wrists, twirl your tongue around their fingers from top to bottom, and breathe over their tummy.

When you eventually arrive between their legs, breathe warm air over them as you skip their genitals (we'll get there soon) and play with their thighs. Move purposefully down their legs, all the way to their toes, and follow your natural inclinations. You can pick up the pace and the pressure as you come back up to their genitals and move on to a more erotic touch—with your hands, lips, tongue, and toys.

Choose any approach that appeals to you as you take their arousal to the next level. We offer a very wide range of oral and manual techniques in the next two chapters, but you can touch, suck, ride, stroke, or vibe in any way that works for you.

A note for the receiving partner: Breathe deeply as your lover touches your body and allow your breath to spread across your body. Pay attention to their touch, tuning into the pressure, speed, rhythm, movement, and temperature. Enjoy the pleasure without concern of reciprocation. Indulge in the connection and give yourself permission to let go of any worries or responsibilities. If allowing your mind to wander into fantasy territory helps you to relax and tune into the sensations, do so without inhibition. If any type of touch feels uncomfortable or bothersome, share your feelings with your partner (with your words, sounds, hands, or movements) so that they can adjust accordingly.

Full-body orgasm is an experience—not a goal. Allow yourselves to indulge in a head-to-toe caress without the pressure to respond in one specific way. You are likely to find that this type of buildup leads to more powerful orgasmic sensations that spread to multiple regions of the body, but if this is not your experience, do not worry. Enjoy the process along with the pleasure and connection of taking your time to explore and experiment.

If you would like to use an audio guide to walk you through the full-body caress, you can access our online version here: happiercouples.com/bodycaress.

PHYSICAL FOREPLAY:
VULVA VERSION

We've said it before and we'll say it again: oral sex *is* sex. In fact, if you have a vulva, it is some of the most satisfying sex you will ever have. Having said that, the magic you weave with your lips and hands can be considered sexual foreplay or the sexual finale. It can change from day to day, and it is up to you to determine whether you experiment with these techniques to seduce your lover en route to other types of sex or allow the oral seduction itself to be the main act.

Before you dive into techniques to titillate the vulva, get to know the region, as it's likely you've run into a good deal of misinformation regarding the vagina, vulva, and clitoris.

For example, we often confuse or conflate the vagina and the vulva, but the **vulva** refers to everything on the outside, and the **vagina** is on the inside.

The vulva includes the outer lips, inner lips, clitoral glans/head, clitoral hood, vestibule, urethral opening, vaginal opening, and mons/pubic mound.

The vagina is a tubelike structure that leads to the uterus via the cervix. Its muscular complex can expand to accommodate objects, but in a resting state, its walls may touch; it is not a gaping hole or tunnel, but a potential space.

Outer lips: You might see diagrams referring to the outer lips as the *labia majora*, but they are not always larger than the inner lips (referred to as the *labia minora*). They run vertically along the border of the left and right sides of the vulva from just above the perineum all the way up to the pubic bone. Hair may grow on them, and they are comprised of both erectile tissue and sensitive nerve endings.

Inner lips: These lips tend to be thinner and hairless, appearing in many shapes, colors, lengths, and sizes. They also extend from top to bottom, covering and providing protection to the vulval vestibule, the vaginal entrance, and the urethral meatus (pee hole).

Vestibule: If you open the inner lips, you will find the **vulval vestibule**, which is a shiny area where you will also find the pee hole (urethral meatus) and entrance to the vagina. The outer edges of this region are referred to as Hart's line, and the U-spot refers to an upside-down U around the urethral opening; both can be to be sensitive to gentle touch (e.g., the tip of a tongue or toy).

The **Bartholin's glands** are two small glands located near the bottom of the vulva, with ducts on either side of the vaginal opening. They are located under the skin, and they can produce a small amount of fluid to lubricate the vulva.

Fourchette: This is the fork in the road at the very bottom where the lips converge together. We often refer to this as the lower clitoris—though it is not officially part of the clitoris. The *fourchette* (French for fork) can be intensely responsive to both light touch (e.g., the flick of a tongue) and firm pressure (e.g., with the pleasure-air tip of the Womanizer).

Pubic mound: At the very top of where the inner and outer lips meet, you will find the fatty skin of the pubic mound where the hair grows. When you rub or grind against this area, it can pull on the foreskin/hood of the clitoris to stimulate the shaft on the inside.

Below the pubic mound, at the top of the vulva, you will find the **clitoral hood** (foreskin), which covers and protects the head (glans) of the clitoris. Often referred to as *the* clitoris, the **head of the clitoris** is a little pea-size nodule that is rich in nerve endings. It is connected to the internal clitoral shaft by a small notch of skin called the frenulum.

The **clitoral shaft** is attached to the clitoral glans and contains erectile tissue, which engorges with blood during arousal, resulting in clitoral boners. The **legs and bulbs/vestibules** of the clitoris are internal components that also swell with pleasure when aroused. The bulbs lie beneath the lips, and the legs extend into the body, pointing toward the thighs when unaroused and stretching back while erect, allowing the clitoris to double in size. The engorgement of the bulbs can cause the vulva to swell and expand outward, which can create a tightening sensation around the outer third of the vagina, which is sometimes referred to as the vagina's *orgasmic platform*.

Because most of us have never been given a tour of our vulva or vagina, and many of us were never even told that the clitoris exists, you may not be familiar with the appearance and location of these beautiful parts. It's time to change this and really get to know the vulva. If you've got your own mirror (or a lover who is willing to give you a tour with theirs), use a hand mirror or sit in front of a full-length wall mirror with your legs apart. Use your fingers to touch your lips. Spread them open, feel their texture, and explore in between them.

Use two hands to open up your inner lips and you will reveal the vestibule, which appears shiny; this is where you will find the entrance to your vagina and urethra. Pull up on the skin at the top of your lips and take a look at the clitoral head, which is round and sometimes looks a little shiny. It may protrude from underneath the hood on its own, or you may need to gently retract the skin to find it. Every clitoris is different, and yours is perfect the way it is.

The vulva and vagina can be positioned at a variety of angles: you might notice that yours is more front facing, midfacing, or back facing. To identify which one you have, stand in front of a mirror. If you can see your vulva or a predominant slit, you likely have a more front-facing vulva. Another way of knowing if you have a front-facing vulva is if you're a person who likes to masturbate on your stomach and/or hump pillows (and other things!). Most people who have front-facing vulvas tend to enjoy these types of sexual activities. If you have a more back-facing vulva, when you're standing in front the mirror you will see mostly the pubic mound, and you might not have a view of the slit or outer lips. Most people who have more predominantly back-facing vulvas and vaginas tend to masturbate on their backs. To maximize sexual satisfaction for back–facing vulvas, try using a pillow or two to lift up off the bed (or other flat surface) so that it's easier to reach your more pleasurable zones. For those of you who have midfacing vulvas and vaginas, you can usually go either way, so lucky you!

No two vulvas are alike, and when it comes to your lips, a range of colors, shapes, thicknesses, and lengths are the norm. If you've been exposed to messages of shame related to your body, you may be uncomfortable with its appearance at first, but research suggests that simply *looking* at your vulva can improve how you feel about your body and that self-exams are also associated with better sexual and overall health. So put down this book and go explore your beautiful self!

Inside the vagina, you will feel the warmth and (possible) wetness of the vaginal canal. With a fairly smooth interior, the vaginal walls contain a limited number of nerve endings, which evolutionary researchers suggest may limit the pain of childbirth (which raises the question as to whether any of these researchers have given birth via the vaginal canal, but that is an entirely different discussion). Despite the fact that the walls contain fewer nerve endings than the clitoris, several spots may produce pleasurable sensations.

The **G-spot** is not a specific spot, but an area that is accessible through the upper wall of the vagina toward the stomach wall. This shallow zone just beyond the vaginal entrance is not a distinct anatomical entity but a series of many sensitive nerve pathways, tissues, and organs that can be felt through the upper wall of the vagina. It often feels different from the rest of the vaginal canal and is described as more ridge-like and textured; some folks say that it feels similar to the roof of your mouth, but softer. Remember, it's usually located between 10 and 2 (like on a clock or driving position), so make sure that you take the opportunity to feel where your perfect time is located.

If you reach in to try to locate the G-spot right now, you may not feel anything remarkable, as you are not aroused. As you stimulate the area and blood flows to the genital region, the tissue begins to swell, and researchers believe that its sensitivity is connected to stimulation of the vaginal[†] prostate, urethral sponge, and inner clitoris.

Exploring a little deeper, beyond the G-spot, you will find the **A-spot** at the back of the upper vaginal wall. Located in the space between the upper wall and the cervix, the A-spot refers to the anterior fornix erogenous zone. Anecdotal reports suggest that this area is associated with rapid lubrication and it can be very sensitive to pressure, so you may want to wait until you

---

[†] Folks of all genders can have vulvas and vaginas. We use "vaginal prostate" rather than "female prostate" to reflect the terminology used in anatomical research while modifying the term out of respect for our audiences and our own sexual politics. Note that the G-spot is not *inside* of the vagina but can be felt through its upper wall.

are highly aroused before touching this area; as arousal builds, the pituitary gland is activated and increased levels of dopamine, endorphins, and oxytocin can have a palliative effect on the body. This chemical release may explain why sensations or touch that might feel uncomfortable during the very early stages of arousal can feel overwhelmingly pleasurable as sexual excitement builds.

Note that getting wet isn't a circus trick, so experiment with stimulation of the A-spot for your own pleasure and not as a matter of performance. And while you are in there, you can also play with your cervix, which has a unique rubberlike texture that feels more firm than the rest of the vagina; some people say it feels like the tip of your nose. (You are touching your nose now, aren't you? We don't blame you!)

Opposite the A-spot on the lower wall of the vagina at the very back, you will find the **cul-de-sac**. Like the A-spot and the cervix, you will likely find that this sensitive area becomes more sexually responsive as orgasm nears and the deluge of feel-good chemicals overtakes the body. During orgasm, your brain activations are similar to those of a brain on drugs, and research suggests that there is only a 5 percent difference between our brain's observable reaction to sex and heroin.[24] This may explain the sense of euphoria experienced during orgasm, as well as why it can feel uncomfortable to press against the cul-de-sac in an unaroused state, but the same sensations can produce intense pleasure when you are highly aroused.

General Guidelines for Going Down

When it comes to seduction, foreplay, and sex, there are no sure-fire moves that will launch every lover's pleasure to new heights, as desires vary not only between lovers, but from day to day. What feels great on a Saturday morning may be off-putting on a Friday night, so you will always be learning and experimenting, and this is what keeps sex fun and exciting in the long run.

If you want to seduce with mastery and finesse, you will need to ensure that communication is both open and ongoing. It follows that the tips and techniques below are intended as guidelines and inspiration, as opposed to perfect prescriptions. Some of these approaches may come naturally, but really great lovers know that the learning process is ongoing.

In general, great lovers are made—not born. Almost anyone can learn to perform a specific technique, talk in a tone with language that turns you on, or approach you in a way that excites you. Sex is not that complicated; we've made it complicated by limiting the ways in which we communicate our sexual needs.

Research shows that good sex requires learning and effort. Those who believe in *sexual growth* are better off than those who believe in *sexual destiny*.[25] That is, if you believe that sex involves learning, investment, and effort, you are more likely to have a satisfying sex life—and you are better able to face challenges when they inevitably arise. If you believe fate determines the outcome of your relationship or sex life, then you are less likely to be satisfied.

If you find yourself thinking that you already know it all, it's probably a sign that you could benefit from slowing down and digging a little deeper. Is there something holding you back from admitting that you have something to learn? Are you avoiding a specific approach by claiming mastery and, if so, what is the source of this avoidance? Even if you and your partner are a match from the onset, you can continue to develop and deepen sexual chemistry with your lover(s), so keep an open mind and consider how you can learn from and expand upon the following suggestions.

Take your time. We know you're excited, and that's a good thing! But most of us move more quickly and apply more pressure than we realize when we're excited and aroused. So whatever your inclination is with regard to speed, cut it in half and then consider slowing down even more. One of the best ways to slow down is to begin with your breath. Before you approach your lover, or as you begin to connect physically, try taking a few deep breaths by inhaling through your nose and exhaling through your mouth. Count as you inhale and exhale, and visualize the air moving throughout your body to allow every square inch to be nourished and aroused by the experience.

Please yourself first. You've probably heard that the key to hotter (oral) sex is *enthusiasm*, but how do you ensure that you are *enthusiastic* about any experience? The answer is simple: you enjoy yourself. In the case of sexual seduction and foreplay, you will be most enthusiastic and confident if you are aroused, so let your mind wander to enjoy your wildest fantasies, use your hands to touch yourself, or wear a vibrating toy that gets you all riled up. The more turned on you are, the more pleasure you will both derive from the experience.

Take it easy. The breasts are not bags of sand and the clitoris isn't a doorbell that needs to be pressed over and over again. More importantly, your lover is not going anywhere, so you don't have to grab them or hold on with all your might. Sometimes a barely there touch is the best way to arouse interest and give your lover time to respond to your advances. You might find that using only the backs of your hands for the first few minutes helps you to touch more gently and sensually, or you can opt to use everything but your hands if you tend to get grabby or if your partner asks you to ease up.

Use your entire body. Do not get hung up on the parts that are engaged with their genitals—pay attention to their entire body using *your* entire body. You might press your skin against theirs, kiss with your lips, lick with your tongue, pull them closer with your legs, grind with your hips, draw them in with your breath, or stroke with your fingertips. Whatever you do, try to engage more than one body part at once if your positioning and flexibility allows for it.

Do what you know and do best. When you are trying a new approach or technique, it is not uncommon to become hyper-focused on the new experience (and its perceived outcomes) at the expense of your existing knowledge and experience. But you already know your body and your partner's, so do not ignore your tried-and-true approaches. In fact, whenever you try something new, it can be helpful to begin with your usual or familiar routine and then add the new component once you are already aroused. As the feel-good chemicals flood your body, you will likely feel less inhibited and more comfortable with new approaches, positions, moves, and scenarios.

Let their body be your guide. Follow their lead. If they are lying still, keep your movements subtle and slow. If their hips are barely moving or flowing in slow motion, allow your actions to mirror theirs. As they increase the movement, intensity, and speed, you can follow suit.

Express pleasure profusely. Do not stifle your sounds or hold your breath. We tend to do both of these things when we're nervous, but doing so not only hinders your own sexual response, it can cause your partner to tense up as well. The more relaxed you are, the more their mood will reflect yours, so breathe deeply and allow your sounds of delight to emanate freely. Moan, groan, and let them know just how much you love their body, your connection, and the experience as a whole. And remember that it is not rude to talk with your mouth full in bed.

Get your face wet. Like most people, you have likely learned much of what you know about oral sex from porn. And though porn can be titillating and entertaining, it is shot for *visual* pleasure—not *physical* pleasure. You will often see cunnilingus scenes in which the tongue is clearly visible and there is a good degree of space between the face and the vulva (they even angle their face to the side so the camera can pick up on their facial expressions); this can be pleasurable, but eventually you will want to get your face right in there. It may not make for a great camera shot, but in real life, you don't have to worry about the viewers.

Change positions. Use pillows to prop up your hips, support your back, pad your knees, and take the pressure off your neck. Flip over, roll on your side, get on all fours, or use props (e.g., scarves or restraints) to ensure you do not tire out. And don't be afraid to change things up in the heat of the action if your muscles are sore or you feel uncomfortable; your comfort is of paramount importance, and the more comfortable you are, the more pleasure you will both experience.

A Note On Lube

Lube makes sex wetter, better, hotter, more exciting, and more varied. Your options for kissing, rubbing, stroking, twisting, grinding, positioning, and riding are simply far greater when the slippery stuff is a part of your regular routine. As you read through the upcoming sections, you will quickly realize that almost every technique requires lube—especially if you like to slip, slide, and grip tightly as you play. This applies regardless of gender.

But lube is not just about variety and technique. Research reveals that those who use lube report higher levels of arousal, pleasure, and sexual fulfillment.[26] And data confirms that symptoms of sexual dysfunction are significantly decreased when you add lube to the mix. Gone are the days in which lube was a matter of anatomical necessity or clinical prescription; lovers of all ages, genders, and sexual orientations now embrace lube as an indispensable sexual enhancement.

If you are looking for creative ways to experiment with lube, consider the following:

▶ Look up into your lover's eyes as you warm the lube up between your palms. Rub a few drops on yourself while maintaining eye contact and then slather it between their legs.

▶ Polish your lips with lube and then use your lips to spread it across their body, beginning with their inner thighs.

▶ Use a soft paintbrush or makeup brush to sensually apply lube or massage oil to your lover's body while they are blindfolded.

▶ Cover your breasts in lube and slide your slippery boobies across their body.

▶ Squeeze some lube into the palm of your hand. Allow it to drip generously onto their skin while you make a show of admiring every square inch.

▶ Put your lubricant in the refrigerator for an hour and apply it with the warm palms of your hands.

▶ Use your breath to warm the lube in your hand before painting it onto your lover's skin.

▶ Institute a no-hands rule when it comes to applying lube so that you will get creative with other props and body parts.

▶ If you have a squeeze bottle, apply it long-distance by holding it up really high and watching it drip down onto your lover's body.

▶ Drip lube into your mouth right before you use it for oral sex!

▶ Use lube shooters during the seduction phase right before (hopefully) sex, and put it in the holes that you anticipate using so they are already good to go.

Clitoral Oral Sex Hacks

Since we know that every vulva is different, it's safe to assume that every clitoris also has its differentiation. These oral sex hacks are perfect depending on the clitoral size and shape.

Round Clitoris = Round Tongue

When you're engaging with a clitoris that is round at the tip, it's often best to use the point of your tongue. Engaging your pointy tongue in circles around the clitoris or in up-down or side-to-side motions can be quite stimulating and a favorite go-to move.

Flat Clitoris = Flat Tongue

If the clitoris in front of you has more of a flat shape to it, using the flat area of your tongue tends to feel phenomenal. Licking in upward motions, or moving your body so that it's perpendicular to their body while licking the clitoris in an upward motion, can get folks who have a more flat clitoris to orgasm.

Small Clitoris = Small Circles | Large Clitoris = Large Circles

If you have a smaller clitoris in front of you (it can be as small as small bead), you can trace around the clitoris using small circles. If there is a larger clitoris in front of you (it can be as big as your thumb), use much larger circles as you work your way around the clitoris.

When it comes to people's differences, smaller clitorises tend to love more pressure and large ones tend to love more sucking. Pay attention to see how large the clitoris gets when it's aroused, because sometimes you may need to move from giving it more pressure to sucking for more pleasure. And of course, pay close attention to your lover's feedback, as they know their body best and these are simply general guidelines.

Now that you are well lubricated and familiar with our general recommendations, we can get down to the nitty-gritty. If you're still here, chances are you are already exceptional in bed. You have embraced the growth mindset and you are a lifelong learner, so you are well on your way to mastering seduction, foreplay, and more. In the next section, we cover a range of techniques and moves you can use to tease, tantalize, and satisfy your lover(s). Feel free to read through the entire lot and then experiment with a few tonight, or highlight the parts that appeal to you and share them with your partner(s). Alternatively, you might opt to open the book to a random page and agree to explore one technique together right now.

We've broken each technique down step by step, but you do not have to follow the directions sequentially. Read through them for inspiration, make adjustments as you see fit, and experiment with ways to improve upon them. You may even want to rename them so that they are more appealing and memorable. Ask your partner(s) for feedback to make them your own.

The V

This smooth and sensuous technique provides pleasure to the full clitoris, including the erectile tissue of its inner components, as you slip and slide along the full length of the vulva.

Play by play:

▸ Slather your hand in your favorite lubricant; with a flat palm, spread your index and middle fingers apart to form a V shape.

▸ Rest your hand over the vulva and slide up and down while you open and close the V formation with your fingers. Move slowly, stroking only once per second.

▸ Begin by hovering your hand over the surface of the lips so that you are barely touching; this allows you to build desire and anticipation while teasing and piquing their interest.

▸ Gradually increase the pressure, following their lead and allowing them to press against you to indicate just how much pressure they desire.

Tantalizing Tip: You can also slip and slide with your hand in a W formation or keep your fingers outstretched in a high-five arrangement. As long as you are sensuously stroking the full length of the lips, you will be stimulating the erectile tissue of the inner clitoris.

The V Cup

Build excitement, anticipation, and pleasure and create an intimate connection by wrapping your hands right around the entire vulva. As you pulse, grind, and undulate, you will pleasure the entire clitoral complex and provide a firm surface against which your lover can bump and grind their way to toe-curling orgasms.

Play by play:

▸ Rest the palm of your hand on the pubic mound. This soft patch of skin (often covered in hair) is oft neglected, but it has the potential to produce a powerful sexual response; when you pull or tug on this area, you retract the hood (or foreskin) of the clitoris, which can create a stroking or rubbing sensation—like a little hand job for the erectile clitoral shaft beneath the hood!

▸ With your palm on the pubic mound, fold your fingers over the entire vulva. You can do this when they are fully dressed, through their underwear, or against their bare skin. If they are naked, you will definitely want to use lube to enhance the sensations.

▸ Once your hand is wrapped around the entire vulva and pubic mound to create your *V cup*, you can press and hold to create warmth and connection. This might be all you do if you are out for dinner or in the car and just looking to build anticipation for what's to come. Alternatively, you can rub, grind, and slide your hand up and down or side to side to stimulate the bulbs of the clitoris via the lips. You might want to undulate your hand in a wavelike motion or pulse to create heat, and you can allow your lover to press and grind according to their preferences.

Tantalizing Tip: Wrap your hand around to create the *V cup* and open up your index and middle finger so that you can slide your tongue, a toy, or another finger inside. Alternatively, use a flat toy like the We-Vibe Wish or the Leaf Fresh in between your fingers and their vulva.

Full-Body Kiss

When you kiss, you experience a rush of feel-good chemicals that promote bonding and relaxation, and kissing is believed to be a gauge of compatibility via the olfactory system. Oral sex is an extension of the lip lock and can create an even more intense reaction as you connect physically and emotionally via a sex act that balances both power and vulnerability.

Play by play:

▶ Begin with gentle kisses over the neck and collarbone, and work your way to one another's lips to kiss passionately as a preview of what's to come.

▶ As you kiss, caress one another's bare skin beneath your clothes, touching with your playful fingertips and warm palms.

▶ Work your way down your lover's body, planting kisses over their collarbone, chest, sides, stomach, and hips. When you arrive between their legs, breathe warm air around the entire area.

▶ Lick up and down their thighs, allowing your cheeks to get wet as they rub against their moistened skin.

▶ With your soft tongue, draw wide ovals over their entire vulva, sweeping around with barely there pressure, and then lick up and down the center of their lips.

▶ Sweep your tongue from side to side before opening wide and kissing their lips with your lips, tongue, and face as though you are French kissing between their legs.

- Suck, slurp, and kiss with enthusiasm as you exude desire with your sounds and body language.

- Do not forget to use your hands as you kiss. Wrap them around their thighs, trace them around their lower back, or slide them beneath their butt cheeks to pull them in close.

Tantalizing Tip: Try this one upside-down to vary the sensations. Straddle your lover's hips and bend over to give them a rear view. They can use their fingers or a toy to impart mutual pleasure.

The Rub-Off

Grinding and rubbing are common paths to orgasm for many folks with vulvas who lie on their stomachs and use a vibrator, bedsheet, pillow, or hand to rub themselves. You can get in on the action and seduce your lover from behind before rubbing them off.

Play by play:

- Ask your lover to lie on their stomach; this position allows them to use their body weight to create extra friction.

- Straddle atop so you can offer a sensual back rub with your favorite massage oil to help you both connect and relax.

- Work your way all around their lower back, neck, and sides, and feel free to turn around to stroke their legs.

- Once you are both in the mood, slide one hand under their mons and allow your lover to rub and grind against it. Follow their movements to determine how much pressure and friction to create.

▸ Kiss their shoulder blades and the small of their back from behind while you rub them off.

While we almost always recommend a generous serving of lube, you may prefer to cut back for this technique to create a bit more friction against the lips and mons.

Tantalizing Tip: Your lover can cross their legs to heighten the sensations of their pelvic floor muscles as your slide your fingers in between and feel their lips swell with pleasure.

Hands-Free Pleasure

Get creative and be playful as you caress your lover's body with everything but your hands.

Play by play:

▸ Use your lips, tongue, breath, forearms, cheeks, chin, hair, chest, legs, and even your toes to explore your lover's body. Blindfold them so that they can home in on the physical sensations and sounds of your approach.

▸ Kiss their collarbone and work your way down their arms. Explore the sides of their chest—you might use a sheet to trace over this area or lick a wet path and breathe over it with warm air.

▸ Pay extra attention to the inner thighs, backs of the knees, small of the back, earlobes, and cheeks—or any other body part that you've yet to explore.

▸ Focus on your own pleasure, too, by rubbing yourself against their supple skin in any way that feels good for you.

▸ Like with each of these techniques, there is no right or wrong way to touch your lover, as long as you've tuned in to their unique responses and you heed their feedback.

Tantalizing Tip: Use props from around the bedroom to create unique sensations. Emery boards can feel a little rough against their legs, while a silk scarf against the nape of their neck might pique their interest. Other household items that can be used for sensual touch include paper clips, spatulas, belts, pillows, stockings, plastic wrap, makeup/shaving brushes, and more. There is no limit to where your imagination can take you.

Double the Pleasure

Play out the fantasy of multiple lovers by simulating a second tongue with the tip of your lubed-up pinkie finger.

Play by play:

▸ Blindfold your lover and warm up your hands so that your finger will feel like a tongue. Because your mouth maintains an average temperature of 98.2 degrees Fahrenheit and your hands likely average approximately 86 degrees, you will need to rub them together or rinse them under hot water if you really want your pinkie finger to feel like a tongue.

▸ Warm up your lover with kisses around their inner ankles, working your way up their inner calves. As you kiss with wet lips, "lick" all around in swerving patterns using a lubed-up pinkie (and ring finger if you prefer) to create the sensation of multiple tongues.

▸ Use your finger(s) and tongue to stimulate their inner thighs and lips.

▶ Breathe generously and stroke between their inner and outer lips using two "tongues."

▶ Stroke up and down the entire length of the vulva with a wet palm so that the sensations are unpredictable and overwhelming.

▶ Add a third "tongue" by using both hands and your tongue simultaneously. Alternate between quick short licks and long, passionate strokes.

Tantalizing Tip: Tease your lover with a little dirty talk. Ask them if they want to be shared. Beg them to let you share and bring another lover in to please and tantalize them. Reinforce the fantasy of multiple tongues by asking them if they like the feeling. Tell them to imagine two (or three) tongues working them from head to toe and heeding their every carnal desire.

My Favorite Toy

Giving oral pleasure offers the unique experience of experimenting with both dominance and submission, as both the giver and receiver. When you go down on your lover, you are often physically positioned in a subservient role (i.e., at their feet), but you wield the power of your mouth and your teeth against their most sensitive skin. In playing the role of My Favorite Toy, you seduce your lover by handing them the reins of control, which not only assuages any performance pressure you might experience, but allows you to enjoy the power and pleasure of submission.

Play by play:

▶ Help your lover to get comfortable sitting on their bum.

Have them lean back with their legs open like a butterfly; the soles of their feet can touch while their knees open and fall to the side.

▶ Lie on your stomach between their legs, adding a pillow for support as needed.

▶ Take their hand and place it on the back of your head so that they can move it around for their own pleasure as they would their favorite toy.

▶ Ask them simple yes or no questions and oblige their every request:

- *More tongue?*

- *Softer? Harder?*

- *Slower? Faster?*

- *Do you like that?*

- *Should I suck more? Lick more? Kiss more?*

▶ Alternatively, you can play with teasing and deprivation with language similar to:

- *Tell me you like it, or I won't let you finish.*

- *I'm going to make you come, but only if you promise to do something for me . . .*

- *I want to hear you scream, or I'll stop and make you wait for it.*

- *Be good and sit on my face, or I'll stop right now and you won't get to finish.*

Teasing with the promise of rewards and denial can activate the pleasure centers of the brain. And as you relinquish control, you are not just playing with power, but building and tapping into the trust you've established in the relationship. Exercising control and power is part of a consensual game underscored by mutual and enthusiastic consent.

And remember that these foreplay approaches are not one-shot deals. You've never really *mastered* a sexual technique or experience, as each encounter will be different depending on your moods, energy levels, and the way you are feeling in your bodies at any given time.

The Thirsty Lover

If you want to turn your lover on and prime them to respond favorably to your advances, be sure to let them know that you crave them—in every way. You want to touch them. You want to taste them. You want to lick them. You want to kiss them. You want to soak them in from head to toe. You can use The Thirsty Lover to entice them as you get warmed up or to finish them off—it is up to you.

Play by play:

▸ Carry or lead your lover to bed and have them sit back against the headboard with their legs bent. Prop their bum up with a few pillows to make it easier to access their hottest spots.

▸ Tuck your head between their thighs and curl your tongue all around. Lick, suck, slurp, and inhale deeply to express your desire and pleasure.

▸ After a few minutes of paying attention to their inner thighs, curl your tongue into the very bottom of the vulva, licking in a scooping motion as though you are soaking up water from a bowl.

▸ Begin with slow, steady licks and work your way up to the clitoris. Lick all around the top of the vulva and rub your face against the mons (pubic mound). Exaggerate your breath as you inhale and soak the area with your kisses.

▸ As your lover's arousal levels increase, speed up your licks until your tongue is fervently lapping up their juices with several licks per second.

Tantalizing Tip: As orgasm approaches, the head of the clitoris can become too sensitive to handle licking, sucking, and direct contact, so pay attention to your lover's reaction and adjust your movements and focus accordingly. Remember that the clitoris is homologous to the penis, so sucking on the head of the clitoris alone is comparable to sucking *only* on the head of the penis and ignoring the rest of its highly responsive parts.

The Thumb Slide

This technique allows you to slip and slide up and down the entire vulva using your thumbs on either side of your tongue. You will provide stimulation to the inner bulbs of the clitoris (through the lips), the fourchette at the base of the lips, and the clitoral hood and head at the top.

Play by play:

▸ Slather your thumbs in your favorite lube and slide them slowly between the inner and outer lips in an up-and-down motion.

▸ Use your tongue in the middle of your fingers (right between the inner lips), licking in the opposite direction.

▸ While you slide your thumbs up between the lips, lick down from top to bottom with the underside of your tongue.

▶ While you slide your thumbs down between the lips, lick up from bottom to top with the tip or body of your tongue.

Tantalizing Tip: Use your wet nose instead of your tongue to slide between their inner lips. Make noise and inhale deeply with every stroke so your lover knows you are enjoying yourself.

Hot and Cold

Play with temperature to launch oral pleasure to new heights, as the tingly sensations amplify pleasure and sexual response around your most delicate and responsive spots.

Play by Play:

▶ Place a glass of ice water and a cup of peppermint tea (or plain hot water) next to your bed.

▶ Begin by breathing warm and cool air over their lips and clit without making physical contact with your mouth. A wide-open mouth will create a warm sensation, while tightly pursed lips will produce cooler air.

▶ Take a sip of water and tuck a small ice cube into your cheek as you begin licking, slurping, and kissing all around. Do not place the ice cube directly on their skin, but allow it to cool your lips, tongue, and cheeks.

▶ After a few minutes, heat things up by taking a sip of the hot tea before you dive back in and resume your sucking, smooching, and stroking. Continue to take quick sips to maintain the heat (use your fingers when you pull away to take a drink), and breathe over the wet spots to make them quiver with delight.

▶ Dip your hands in the cool water before playing with

your lover's nipples or running a few fingers over their backside.

Tantalizing Tip: Add a little amaretto, rum, or bourbon to your mint tea or use a mint-flavored breath strip to heighten the tingle.

Be Still My Hart

Hart's line refers to the path that surrounds the sensitive vestibule of the vulva. The vestibule is the shiny section between her inner lips and is the site of the glands associated with lubrication and female ejaculation. Tracing a subtle line around this area with faint touch will likely help your lover to relax and get in the mood for more and more pleasure.

Play by play:

▶ Wrap your arms around your lover and kiss their neck and ears before kneeling at their feet.

▶ Help them to sit comfortably on the edge of a chair, couch, or bed and caress their legs while undressing them.

▶ Use the backs of your fingers to very gently trace curvy lines over their inner thighs. Kiss the backs of their knees and allow your cheeks to brush between their legs and against their warm lips.

▶ Open your mouth wide and breathe warm air all around their thighs, hips, and pubic mound.

▶ Gently peel open their inner labia with your thumbs and use a flat tongue to lick the shiny vestibule from bottom to top as slowly as possible. Slow your pace to one lick every three seconds.

▸ Twirl your tongue around the fourchette (the delicate spot at the bottom of where the labia meet).

▸ When they start squirming with delight, trace the tip of your tongue around the outer edge of the vestibule to follow Hart's line. Alternate between clockwise and counterclockwise movements and play with speed—move slowly for a few laps and then more quickly, alternating back and forth.

Tantalizing Tip: Throw a bullet vibe like Crave Duet into the mix and trace Hart's line with its precise vibrating tips.

V on the G
Use your fingers to slide along the G-spot while you simultaneously lick the head of the clitoris to send waves of pleasure throughout her body via the vagus and pudendal nerves.

Play by play:

▸ Kneel on the floor at your lover's feet as they lie on the bed with their legs hanging off the edge. Place pillows below your knees and beneath their head for comfort, and encourage them to lie back and relax so you can cater to their every need.

▸ Press your tongue against the very top of the vulva over the hood and head of the clitoris. Lick up and down with warm short strokes, alternating between the top and the underside of your tongue to vary the texture and sensations.

▸ Breathe deeply and slowly as you lick with firm pressure to encourage your lover to slow their breath as well.

▸ Lube up your index and middle fingers and slide them

inside the vagina beneath your tongue. Press them up toward your partner's stomach, against the upper wall. You might feel the ridge-like texture of the G-spot as you press against the upper wall.

▸ Do not stop licking.

▸ With every lick upward, spread your fingers apart to form a peace sign (in a scissor-like motion); with every lick downward, pull your fingers back together.

▸ Continue to lick the clitoris on the outside while sliding your fingers along the inner wall of the vagina to stimulate the G-spot in rhythm with each lick.

Note: You don't want to get hung up on the coordination of your hands and fingers, so if trying to time your finger slides and tongue movements feels distracting or unnatural, try an alternative approach: simply press your tongue against the head of the clitoris while you slide your fingers inside. You likely will not have to move your tongue at all, as your partner's hips will do the rocking and grinding for you.

Tantalizing Tip: Rather than using just your index and middle fingers to form a V, add your ring finger into the mix and open and close to form a W against the upper wall to stimulate the G-spot. And if they prefer vibrations against the clitoris, use a toy that pinpoints the head of the clitoris (check out the We-Vibe Tango or the Womanizer Pro) instead of your tongue. They can hold it in place and you can work your tongue around the lower vulva to lick and suck the sensitive fourchette.

The Voyeur

Use a mirror beside the bed to give your partner a view of the action while you lick, slurp, suck, and breathe it all in between their legs.

Play by play:

▸ Position a mirror next to the bed and have your lover kneel on the bed facing the mirror.

▸ Lie on your back and slide between their legs from behind, with your head toward the mirror and feet pointing away. Pile pillows beneath your head so that you can easily reach their hot spots and your neck is well supported.

▸ Begin by licking around their inner thighs. Get them soaked and let your cheeks swirl all around the wet spots you have created. Breathe it all in and let your lover know that you love the way it feels, tastes, and smells.

▸ Use your nose and the tip of your tongue to softly tease the lips with featherlight pressure.

▸ Stick your tongue out as far as you can and trace it against the lips, leaving enough space for your lover to watch your tongue at play in the mirror. Tease for a while, and when their breath rate begins to quicken, increase the pressure.

▸ Press your lips all around the vulva and suck while you twirl your tongue in all directions.

▸ Use your nose to slide up and down and side to side. Press it in the vagina, against the head of the clitoris, and all around the fourchette.

▸ Use your hands to pull them closer and allow your lips

and fingers to wander, ensuring that they get a full view of the action.

Note: If your partner's knees get sore, they can bend over and rest on all fours. If your neck tires, change positions or add more pillows so that it is fully supported.

Tantalizing Tip: Approach them from behind while they are in front of the mirror. Press your body up against theirs and caress them all over so they can watch. If they are busy (e.g., running off to work), you will be setting the mood for their return, and if they have time to play, you can turn them to the side so they can watch you work your magic.

The Joystick

Allow your lover to take control and use your face, lips, tongue, and more for their ultimate pleasure.

Play by play:

▸ Lead your lover to the edge of the bed. Drop to your knees and help them to undress, removing shoes, pants, skirts, socks, underwear, and anything else from the waist down.

▸ Look up at them and share your own version of "I'm here to cater to your every need."

▸ Add pillows beneath your knees for comfort.

▸ Rest your head on their thighs. Take a few deep breaths here, soaking in everything you feel—the texture of their skin against your cheeks, the temperature and scent of their body, the sounds of the room and your breath.

▸ Place your lover's hands on the back of your head and

tell them to guide you as they like it. They can control the speed, direction, pressure, rhythm, and strokes by directing your head with their hands.

▶ Look up in their eyes and ask if they want it harder, softer, slower, or faster.

▶ Talk with your mouth full to let them know you are enjoying yourself: *I love the way you taste. I want to soak it all in. I want to take care of you however you want it.*

▶ Allow them to control your movements (within your own physical and emotional comfort) and follow their hips as a guide to gauge their desired speed, direction, and pressure.

▶ Breathe deeply and allow your sounds to emanate freely without inhibition; this will encourage your partner to do the same.

Tantalizing Tip: It is perfectly acceptable to talk with your mouth full during oral sex, but if communication becomes stifled, you might want to create a few nonverbal codes to indicate your desires when you cannot speak. For example, a squeeze of the hand might indicate that you want your partner to slow down, and two taps might indicate that you want more pressure. Negotiate these communication codes in advance, and once you become accustomed to using them during sex, you can play with them outside the bedroom to tease and build tension throughout the day/week.

Twirl and Suck

Overwhelm your lover with pleasure using your lips, tongue, breath, and suction. This technique allows you to stimulate the entire vulva from the lips (and inner clitoral bulbs) to the sensitive head of the clitoris and the responsive fourchette—this area is packed with erogenous tissue and thousands of nerve endings.

Play by play:

▸ Look your lover up and down from head to toe. Admire every inch of their body as you smile and lower your eyes. Kiss all around their stomach, hips, thighs—start light and gentle, and increase the intensity over the course of several minutes.

▸ Before you dive down between their legs, look up at them and hold the eye contact for a few extra seconds.

▸ Open your mouth and stick out your tongue. Turn from side to side as though you are shaking your head no, and move up and down as though you are nodding yes. Lick around with the tip of your tongue to rile them up.

▸ Once their arousal builds, open your mouth as wide as you can to cover the entire length of their beautiful vulva. Suck with your lips as you twirl your tongue around the inner perimeter of your mouth. Allow the sucking sounds to flow freely as you continue to suck and twirl—changing directions and flicking against the head of the clitoris and the delicate fourchette.

▸ Keep the suction cup of your lips constant as you twirl your tongue around the entrance of the vagina. Increase the speed and pressure in response to the movement of their hips.

Tantalizing Tip: Keep your hands engaged while your mouth is busy between their legs. Wrap your hands around their butt to pull them closely into your face or slide up and fondle their nipples. Better yet, reach down and touch yourself—the more turned on you are, the more you will enjoy your lover's pleasure, and vice versa.

Pleasure Pulse

Pulsing sensations not only mimic the sensation of orgasmic contractions, but they can trigger, prolong, and intensify orgasms. By pulsing against various body parts that you may not associate with orgasm, you can also learn to experience orgasmic pleasure across the body.

Play by play:

- ▶ Lower the lights and crawl into bed, assuming a spooning position with your lover as the small spoon.

- ▶ Kiss their neck and play with their hair/scalp from behind.

- ▶ Use flat palms in large sweeping motions across their back, and trickle your fingers gently across their under-arms and the sides of their chest as you work your way down.

- ▶ Wrap your arms around them and place your hand around their labia to envelop the entire vulva. Rub up and down. Slide your fingers inside.

- ▶ Use your other hand to caress their skin as their arousal builds.

- ▶ Use your lips to create heat against their backside.

- ▶ Once their breath rate increases and their hips are moving more quickly and powerfully, pulse your hand over the entire length of their lips, or press two fingers over the head of the clit and pulse.

- ▶ If you can reach around with both hands, you can slide a few fingers inside and pulse against the roof of the vagina while you simultaneously pulse your other hand on the outside.

▶ Or, you might use your other hand to pulse against other erogenous zones across the full body, such as the neck and shoulders, the belly button, the nipples, or the perineum.

▶ You can pulse more slowly at first, and then pick up the pace to one to two pulses per second, continuing to pulse as they orgasm.

Tantalizing Tip: Rather than approaching from behind, you can climb between their legs and use your tongue, lips, and toys to mimic the contractions of orgasm. When you pulse against their hot spots, they may subconsciously recall the physical experience of orgasm, including the muscular spasms felt in the entire pelvic region and beyond. Because orgasmic sensations are not limited to the genitals (some people feel it in their belly button, their lower back, their hips, and even their cheeks), do not limit your pulsing to the clitoris or vagina alone.

You can add a pulse to any move, technique, or position:

▶ Pulse your lips against the entire vulva.

▶ Slide your thumb over the head of the clitoris and pulse with deep pressure.

▶ Press two fingers along the perineum and pulse every half second.

▶ Gently pinch and release their nipples between your thumb and middle finger.

▶ Pulse your index and middle fingers against their pucker (the butt hole).

▶ Pulse in an undulating motion as you cup your hand around the entire vulva.

▶ Curl two fingers or a toy against the G-spot and pulse and release.

Fingers Crossed

There are countless ways to use your hands to seduce and tantalize your lover, and the fingers-crossed approach is one of our favorites. With a subtle shift to your traditional fingering technique, you will create new and unique sensations to excite your lover with the unexpected.

Play by play:

▶ Have your lover get on all fours or lie on their back, front, or side with their legs open. Any position will work, so just ensure that you are both comfortable.

▶ Begin with some warm circular strokes against their butt cheeks or thighs, and lay on the compliments with whatever comes to your mind. Just be sure to let them know how much you admire their every curve.

▶ Cross your index and middle fingers and cover them in lubricant.

▶ Gently insert your fingers inside and rotate from the wrist as you slide in and out.

▶ Move more slowly than you might naturally be inclined to at first so that you can increase the speed as their arousal heightens. If you can, look them in the eye, smile, and let them know how much you delight in their pleasure.

Tantalizing Tip: As they become more aroused, you can broaden your rotations to scoop a little wider against the inner walls of the vagina—pay attention to their bodily movements and facial expressions to ensure that the pressure is just right. If you have a spare hand, play with their hips, clit, nipples, butt, or yourself!

The Nose Job

The most memorable and generous lovers know that sex can get a little messy and more than a little wet, and they are not afraid to mess up their hair or makeup. Use your entire face to get your lover off by giving them a nose job and more.

Play by play:

▸ Lie on your lover's stomach or position yourself between their legs so that you can seduce them with a sensual massage of their legs. Trace your finger tips in s-l-o-w figure eights over the full surface of their ankles, calves, and thighs (or wherever you can reach from your current position). Use your palms to stroke in ovals and create some heat as you incidentally brush against their hotter spots to tease and build desire. If you can, use your cheeks and nose to caress their legs, working your way from the outer sections to the inner thighs. Slow and deepen your breath as you explore their body.

▸ Once you are both feeling relaxed, trace a wet line from the very base of the vulva (try to get all the way down to their perineum or fourchette) all the way up to their mons using a flat, wide tongue, ensuring that you leave a warm path behind. Slide the tip of your nose from top to bottom along the wet path you've created, and then come back up the middle, breathing warm air along the same wet path. Repeat as you lick to create a wet spot and then roll the tip of your nose down the wet spot.

▸ Lick, kiss, suck, slurp, slide, and stroke to your heart's delight.

▸ As their arousal heightens, they'll need something to grind against. And that *something* is your face. Get your nose in there and rock back and forth, up and down, and around in sensual ovals. Slide the tip of your nose right inside the vagina, allowing their lips to rub and grind against your cheeks.

▸ Press your nose against the clit and slide your hands behind them to pull them in closer. Encourage them to wrap their legs right around your head.

▸ Breathe deeply through your mouth so that you can bury your nose and allow them to ride it all the way to orgasm.

Tantalizing Tip: If they enjoy the Nose Job, use the tip of your nose to remind them of the experience and build tension at unpredictable moments. Run the tip of your nose against the back of their neck while they are at the computer, or nuzzle your nose against their neck and ears as you're snuggling on the couch watching a movie.

Pinch and Screw

This move has it all: fingering the G-spot, playing with the external clit, and tonguing the fourchette and orgasmic platform.

Play by play:

▸ Kneel at your lover's feet while they sit on the edge of the bed or a chair. Alternatively, they can lie on their back and you can straddle them at the chest facing their feet.

▶ Begin by slathering both hands in lube and giving your lover a thigh job. Slide your wet fingers, palms, and the backs of your hands all around their thighs. Add your lips and tongue into the mix, and allow them to hover over their labia without touching, so that they are aching for more of your touch.

▶ Slide your index and middle fingers inside their vagina and press up toward the G-spot; press your thumb against the outer clitoris and pinch gently so that you are pinching as you slide out and releasing as you insert.

▶ Angle your fingers to accommodate your tongue sliding into the vagina beneath them. Continue the pinching motion with your fingers as you slide your tongue all around—you can screw in and out or simply roll it around to feel the warmth and to taste everything your lover has to give.

Note: Because this technique requires some maneuvering and coordination, adjust it so that it feels natural for you. The last thing you want to be thinking about is technique when you are enjoying your lover's body, so consider these moves as inspiration, but don't allow them to overtake the experience. If at any point you feel distracted, take a big deep breath in through your nose and pay attention to everything you smell; as you exhale, smile and take note of the physical sensations throughout your body, using your senses to bring you back to the present moment.

Up and Down
For this technique, play with power and build tension by delaying orgasm with simple positional changes. Alternate between riling them up into a preorgasmic delirium and then bringing them back down with gentle caresses. Rinse and repeat until you

are both ready to explode. Begin with a full-body caress set to candlelight, using oil, warm breath, and the soft touch of your lips and fingertips.

Play by play:

▶ Sweep your lover off their feet and help them get comfortable lying on their back with a pillow beneath their head and knees. Block out visual distractions with a scarf or eye mask and begin with a full-body caress. Work your way from top to bottom and bottom to top, drawing your focus and energy to their hips. Use a variety of strokes and vary your pressure, paying attention to the feeling of their skin beneath your fingertips. Use the soft pads of your fingers, the warm touch of your palms, as well as your lips and breath to explore the entire surface of their body.

▶ Once you can feel their body relaxing into the pleasure of your touch, slide your hands beneath them and turn them over to lie facedown with the pillow under their hips.

▶ Spread their legs and dive in from behind, eating, sucking, and soaking it all in with ravenous desire. Squeeze their inner lips together between your lips, and run your tongue in the groove.

▶ Stick your nose between their legs and rub it around in every direction while your hands grab their bum cheeks and massage with passion.

▶ Slide your fingers inside and twirl gently as you suck on the outside, allowing your slurps and moans to radiate across your bodies.

▶ When you feel their hips gyrating with greater intensity

and you sense that their arousal is building, slide your hands beneath their thighs and guide them onto their back once again.

▶ Gently caress the outer edges of their chest, breathe over their nipples, and trickle your fingernails over their mons. Spread your thumbs ever so slowly over their labia, allowing their breath and heart rate to slow as you decrease your speed and pressure. Spend a minute or two here until they've calmed down and their breath rate has slowed.

▶ Once they are nice and calm again, turn them back onto their stomach to dive in once again. Use your tongue to slide back and forth, round and round, and in and out. Breathe in and exhale deeply with pleasure. Use your hands to stroke, your lips to kiss, your tongue to lick, and your face to grind. Rile them into a preorgasmic frenzy, but do not let them go over the edge.

▶ As soon as you sense that they are about to reach orgasm, turn them onto their back again and caress their face, stomach, and thighs until they are begging for more.

▶ Repeat this sequence of offering gentle pleasure while they are on their back and turning up the heat when you flip them onto their tummy.

▶ You may opt to eventually take them over the edge using your oral skills, or you might switch roles or activities according to your preferences.

For the receiver: If you feel an orgasm coming on, let your lover know by allowing your body's natural responses—including sounds, movements, and facial expressions—to flow freely. Encourage your body to release groans, moans, and whimpers and to be vocal throughout the experience so that your lover can accurately gauge your level of arousal.

The Tongue Twister

Your tongue is one of the strongest muscles, so you can use it in almost any way that you use your fingers to make your lover quiver with delight.

Play by play:

▶ Slide your tongue in and out of the vagina, rolling it around to enjoy the warm, soft folds. Alternate between your fingers and tongue to vary the sensations.

▶ Roll your tongue into a tube and slide it over the head of your lover's clitoris. You may need to pull up on the hood to reveal the nerve-rich head, as it can retract beneath the surface as its sensitivity increases.

▶ Roll your tongue into a tube and slide it in and out of the vagina while breathing deeply. To learn to roll your tongue, purse your lips tightly and try to push your tongue out while rolling the sides in toward one another. If you really cannot roll your tongue, fret not! You can pinch the sides of your tongue together with your fingers to create an equally sexy tube.

Tantalizing Tip: While you slide your tongue in and out of the vagina, tickle your nose against the head of the clitoris while you press your lips all around the vulva to create a suction cup.

Inner Peace

Combine the pleasure of clitoral licking and kissing with the power of your fingers to spread the erotic pleasure back to the outer edges of the G-spot. This multiple-area approach can intensify sensations as pleasure signals are relayed to the brain via the pelvic, vagus, and pudendal nerves.

Play by Play:

▸ Kneel at their feet as they lie on the bed with their legs hanging off the edge.

▸ Press your tongue against the very top of the vulva, over the hood of the clit, at the bottom of the Venus mound. Lick up and down with short strokes, alternating between the top and the underside of your tongue to vary the texture and sensations.

▸ Slide your wet index and middle fingers inside with your palm facing up, and press against the upper vaginal wall to feel for the swollen ridges of the G-spot.

▸ Maintaining pressure against the G-spot, spread your fingers apart to form a peace sign and close them rhythmically as though they are a pair of scissors.

Tantalizing Tip: Experiment with varied touch patterns against the G-spot through the vagina. Use three fingers to open and close in the shape of a W, or alternate between spreading your fingers open and swiping them back and forth like a windshield wiper.

Squirter! (The Come Hither)

Ejaculation is not just for penises. Ancient sexuality texts as old as the *Kama Sutra* provide documentation of female ejaculation. Squirter orgasms are associated with G-spot stimulation and often described as unique in terms of the sensation and full-body experience. This makes sense, as the G-spot is believed to communicate with the brain via the vagus nerve, which wanders throughout the body.

Though squirting is not a sideshow trick or a universal sign of a more intense orgasm, you might discover new pathways to pleasure as you explore different types of orgasm. It's important to note that you can ejaculate without having an orgasm, just as you can orgasm without ejaculating. They are two distinct processes for people of all genders, despite the fact that penises tend to ejaculate and orgasm at the same time.

In most cases, the fluid expelled during ejaculation is less than a teaspoon in volume, and unlike the squirting depicted in porn, it doesn't usually spray across the room. Unless you've hidden a SuperSoaker in your vagina, it is often more of a drip or dribble than a visible gush. Of course, there are exceptions to every rule. Some people squirt more and some people squirt less, but the volume of fluid is not an indication of pleasure or sexual prowess. Like sweat and saliva, the amount of fluid produced varies from person to person. You do you, and let others enjoy sex on their own terms.

Research suggests that the skene's glands, which drain into the urethra and are often considered a part of the G-spot, are associated with squirting. Embedded in the spongy tissue that surrounds the urethra, the skene's glands are considered homologous to the prostate gland. If follows that the contents of ejaculate are similar to prostatic fluid and contain prostatic-specific antigen, prostatic acid phosphatase, urea, creatinine, glucose, and fructose.[27] In terms of taste, some describe the fluid as a little sweet, and others say that it has almost no taste at all.

Because of the location of these glands around the urethra, between the vagina and the bladder, pressure in this area—including the G-spot via the upper vaginal wall—can make you feel as though you have to pee. Combined with the fluid expelled, it makes sense that many folks feel self-conscious about squirting, as they are concerned that the fluid expelled may contain urine. In response to this fear, folks might avoid stimulation of this area or tense up to avoid a squirter orgasm altogether.

However, most research suggests that you have nothing to worry about. Not only can you empty your bladder beforehand to alleviate these concerns, but ultimately, if some urine were to be expelled along with the ejaculate, it's no big deal and will likely go unnoticed.

Squirting, like all sex acts, isn't for everyone. Some folks love it and find that squirter orgasms are the most intense and pleasurable. Others, however, find them to be average at best and not worth the extra laundry. Whatever your reaction, you are perfectly normal. Just as some people love a good foot rub and others prefer not to have their feet touched, a range of experiences are healthy, and you do not need to measure yours against anyone else's.

If you do want to explore G-spot and squirter orgasms, consider the Come Hither and allow yourself to enjoy the pleasure of the process as opposed to seeking a specific outcome.

Play by play:

- ▸ Kiss, fondle, and caress your lover's body for a few minutes.

- ▸ Rub, touch, and lick between their legs—against their lips, clitoris, and thighs—until their hips are thrusting and you can hear them breathing deeply.

- ▸ Insert your middle and ring finger into the vagina and curl them up against the upper wall.

- ▸ Alternate between a come-hither motion over the G-spot and a tick-tock movement from side to side with both fingers. You will likely feel the G-spot swell against the wall as the area engorges with blood.

▸ Use your tongue to lick and suck away as you please.

▸ As orgasm approaches, continue to stimulate the G-spot with a come-hither motion as you place your other hand on their lower abdomen. Press and release smoothly in rhythm with your come-hither motion. This will allow you to stimulate the urethral sponge (the site of the G-spot) from both the inside and the outside.

▸ If you'd like to change it up, you can also do the G-Circle. Use your fingers in a circular motion around the G-spot, while simultaneously moving them in and out and firmly pressing up against that ridged tissue.

▸ Alternatively, you can pull your fingers out and stimulate the U-spot by rubbing your index and middle finger on either side of the urethral opening, along the vestibule.

▸ Encourage your lover to breathe deeply and allow the pleasure to overtake their body.

The Self-Service (for Solo G-Spot Play)

Reaching your G-spot with your own hands can be a challenge, but there are many toys on the market designed to stimulate this sensitive area and beyond.

The **We-Vibe Nova** is an updated version of the old-school rabbit vibrators, and its two arms provide dual stimulation to the G-spot internally and to the clitoris externally. Because it stimulates two distinct areas that are believed to communicate with the brain via two separate nerve pathways (the pudendal nerve and the vagus nerve), it has the potential to produce varied and more intense orgasms—including squirter orgasms. The inner arm curves into the vagina to press on the upper wall and stimulate the G-spot with rumbly vibrations, and the outer arm bends to press and vibrate against the hood, shaft, and head of the clitoris on the outside.

When using a toy like the Nova to experiment with G-spot orgasms, experiment with thrusting and rocking motions. Rock back and forth in a circular motion or pulse it against the G-spot to experiment with different rhythmic sensations. You might also try inserting it while you are lying on your side so that you can squeeze your legs together and increase the pressure against your lips (to access the internal bulbs of the clitoris).

The **Womanizer Duo** offers an alternative to vibrators like the Nova, as the outer arm stimulates the head of the clitoris with pleasure-air technology that uses tiny bursts of air to create a suction-like sensation over the head (and shaft) of the external clitoris. The inner arm curves upward against the G-spot to provide vibrations internally, and each function can be controlled individually, so you can customize with gentle suction on the outside and powerful vibrations internally, or any combination of your choosing.

If you prefer direct G-spot stimulation (rather than dual stimulation of the external clitoris), the **We-Vibe Rave** is a good option, as its asymmetrical design makes accessing the G-spot a breeze. Though the Rave appears to be a basic phallus-shaped vibe, it has an ergonomic handle for easy maneuvering as well as soft "pleasure edges" for a little extra stimulation against your most sensitive spots. Try rocking back and forth or side to side and pulsing against the upper inner wall. Start with vibrations beginning at the lowest setting and gradually work your way up (it has ten preset intensities, but you can also create your own vibrations using the We-Connect app). You can also ride the Rave to orgasm using your hips rather than maneuvering it with your hands. Once you are relaxed, hold the Rave steady and work your hips around it as though you are riding it. There is no need to overthink this approach—simply let your hips move in whatever way feels natural and pleasurable.

Should you prefer a smaller model with a flexible tip that you can adjust to suit your individual angles, the **Crave Flex** vibrator is unique, as its functions were uniquely crowdsourced. A community of beta testers helped to design the twelve vibrating settings, and you can bend the soft tip to adjust the pressure against your G-spot.

Use the Crave Flex in the palm of your hand as you rub and grind, or angle it to curl around the entrance of your vagina and against the head of your clitoris.

A note on getting wet: Since we are talking about squirting, we'd be remiss not to talk about other bodily fluids, including vaginal lubrication. Getting wet is often touted as a sign of arousal, but it is important to remember that a wetter reaction is not necessarily a sign of a greater desire for sex, and a dry response does not indicate a lack of interest. Sometimes you are turned on and dry as a desert, and sometimes you are walking down the street wondering why a geyser has sprouted between your legs. This is because our body's physiological reactions to sexual desire and arousal do not always align with our lived experience or our mental arousal, and that's okay. So please do not fret if you don't squirt or get soaking wet during sex—you can always use lube (it makes sex so much better!), and you are not missing out on anything as long as you're enjoying the process and relishing the present moment.

PHYSICAL FOREPLAY:
PENIS PROGRAM

Oh the mighty penis! Honored as the ultimate sex symbol as well as the butt of many jokes, the messages related to the penis are often discordant, and stereotypes abound.

Size, for example, tends to be the focus of unending conversations around virility, sexual prowess, power, confidence, and even stamina. But size is often irrelevant to the way you give and receive pleasure. Bigger is not necessarily better, and a good fit and an open mind will go a great deal farther than an extra inch or two. Just as vaginas, anuses, mouths, and hands vary in size and this does not affect the quality of a sexual relationship, penis size need not determine the quality of a sexual experience or connection.

It is neither the size of the wave nor the specific motion in the ocean that makes for good sex—an open mind and a desire to meet one another's needs outweigh size and enduring stamina.

When you think about penis size—yours and/or your partner's—consider the difference between what turns you on naturally versus what you find attractive and enticing based on cultural norms. Size may matter in terms of cultural expectations, but does it really matter to *you*? If you allow your natural animalistic lust to dictate your desires without regard for what you are *supposed* to want, you will likely find that your tastes are more diverse and your experiences are more fulfilling. If, on the other hand, you seek partners who fit a prescribed norm of beauty, you may find that your connections and experiences are both limiting and disappointing. This is true for penis size as well as other elements of physical, social, and emotional attraction.

As you explore these foreplay techniques, you will note that not only is size mostly irrelevant (aside from finding a comfortable fit in your hands, mouth, vagina, butt, or any other body part you decide to connect with), but hardness is not a prerequisite to pleasure either. **You do not have to have an erection to enjoy sex, and in fact, you do not need a penis to explore these techniques.** If you have a partner who has a strap-on, some of these moves can prove quite useful in your seduction journey. Although many of these approaches cater to those whose partners have penises, do not allow your partner's genitals to limit your pleasure. Regardless of anatomy, experiment with these moves and adjust them to your liking—you will find that many will be a good fit for your favorite phallus of any type.

Before we get started, let us take a tour of the penis and its related parts. Penises come in different shapes, sizes, colors, curves, and thicknesses. Because every penis is unique, you have to treat them differently, exploring diverse approaches to touching, kissing, licking, and stroking.

Now, it's time to get to know the penis from the bottom to the top (literally!).

The **prostate** (or P-spot), which swells during arousal, is often compared to the vagina's G-spot and can be accessed through the **anus**. It is located between the pelvic floor and the bladder, and it is also against the front wall of the anus, with its muscular and glandular tissue surrounding the urethra. It is primarily responsible for helping to carry and sustain sperm and is soft and smooth to the touch. It is not a part of the penis, but an interior neighbor homologous to the vaginal G-spot.

Next up is the **perineum** (commonly referred to as the taint or gooch). This is the area between the anus and the scrotal sac containing fibromuscular tissue that is usually sensitive to touch, pressure, and vibrations. It is also the site of the bulbospongiosus muscle that covers the bulb of the penis and its vessels and nerves. You might be able to recognize the area because it contains less hair than the scrotum and immediate area surrounding the anus.

The bulb of the penis (sometimes referred to as the B-spot) is the sensitive area of the inner penis that you can access through the perineum. Press your fingers, a toy, or your tongue right behind the scrotal sac to stimulate the inner section of the penis, which has been historically referred to as the Million-Dollar Point.

This area tends to be sensitive to touch and pressure, as it includes extensions of the corpora cavernosa, crura, and corpus spongiosum. The corpora cavernosa are two tubelike structures that fill with blood during an erection, and the crura of the penis are homologous to the inner legs of the clitoris. The corpus spongiosum wraps around the urethra, forming the sensitive head of the penis, but also extends all the way down to the bulb. It is covered by the bulbospongiosus muscle.

We often assume that stroking from base to tip covers the entire penis, but if you really want to stimulate the entire organ, you will want to combine your external pleasure with pressure against the internal bulb. MRI images reveal that the penis curves inside the body, forming a shape similar to a boomerang, and many people with penises report that the orgasmic contractions are felt most intensely in the inner bulb.

At the end of the chapter, we'll share a few strategies for stimulating the B-spot and prostate.

Head north of the perineum to run into the scrotal sac (or **scrotum**), containing the testes. It has to maintain a temperature that is cooler than the body to promote sperm production, so the scrotum hangs from the body. When touching them, you may be able to feel the testes along with the extra skin of the scrotal sac.

Extending from just above the scrotum is the **shaft** of the penis. At rest, it is soft and limp, but when engaged (mentally or physically), it can swell with blood and become firm. This firmness is called an erection.

The **raphe** is the dividing line that runs all the way from the anus to the tip of the penis. It traverses the perineum, scrotum, and shaft.

Covering the head of the penis is the retractable and highly innervated **foreskin**. Some people have this skin removed via the process of circumcision. Although the media and porn portray circumcised penises more often, the majority of penises in the world are uncircumcised.

At the top of the shaft is the sensitive **head** of the penis (similar to the head of the clitoris). Filled with thousands of nerves, the spongy tissue swells and surrounds the urethra.

On the underside of the head, you will find the **frenulum**. One of the most important pleasure spots on the penis (and the whole body, at that), it is a sensitive notch that attaches the foreskin to the phallus.

The ridge that surrounds the bottom of the head is called the **corona**, and its circumference is smooth and reactive to touch.

At the very tip of the penis, you will find the **urethral meatus**. This is where urine and semen are expelled—though not simultaneously.

Just the Tips

We know you are ready to dive in headfirst, but before you start sucking and stroking, you will want to seduce your lover by building anticipation and giving them a taste of what's to come.

Pique their interest by *almost* wrapping your hand or hands around the penis or strap-on and keeping your fingers loose while stroking from base to tip.

Press your tongue around the base and lick a slow line up the middle of the shaft, all the way to the tip. Take your time to truly connect with your partner.

Cover the palm of your hand in lube and slide it over their shaft and head in long, sweeping motions. Open your index and middle fingers to slide around the sides and vary the pressure. Do not *grab* it yet, just *slide* around the shaft of the penis! And don't worry about whether or not it is erect. This technique, like most, does not require a hard penis.

Sweep your tongue under, over, and around their balls or perineum as you look up at them longingly.

Roll your tongue all around the shaft to leave a messy wet path, open your mouth wide, and breathe sensual, warm air over the wet spots you've created. Alternate between warm air using a wide-open mouth and cool air, which you can create by pursing your lips as you exhale.

Bear in mind multiple seduction learning styles as you approach with enthusiasm. Think about how you look—from their point of view as well as your own. Consider the sounds you are making as you lick, stroke, and suck. Go out of your way to use a variety of touch techniques that you know your lover adores—as well as new ones that might arouse their curiosity.

As you approach them, do not go to your money moves right away. If you start with The Mind-Blower, you will be giving away the farm from the onset, and you will likely be physically exhausted. Instead, seduce and rile your lover into a frenzy with approaches and techniques intended to pique interest, cultivate anticipation, and allow the sensations of pleasure to spread across the body. Yes—the penis is a hotbed of pleasure, but erotic and orgasmic sensations can be even more powerful when experienced after a buildup of psychological and physical tension.

Speaking of sexual tension, be sure to get yours too. Get yourself turned on so that you will be more relaxed and experience an increase in confidence. If you want to give (and enjoy) a masterful blow job, enthusiasm is key. And what better way to get enthusiastic than to activate your own sexual response cycle? When you are aroused, your inhibitions and self-consciousness often diminish as the pituitary gland, nucleus accumbens, and ventral tegmental areas are activated and the hypothalamus goes into overdrive. The center of reasoning and behavior in the brain shuts down, and the amygdala, which controls emotion, is activated. As your brain and body become awash in an eruption of chemicals, you are likely to be overwhelmed by your own pleasure and more naturally inclined toward sharing it with your partner.

And finally, be sure to use lube. It goes without saying that the majority of these techniques require lube to work—unless you are into penile chafing (in which case, you do you). And even those that do not *require* lube will likely be more comfortable, pleasurable, and easy to perform if you use a few drops of the slippery stuff.

We outline these techniques play by play with Tantalizing Tips to inject variety and enhance pleasure. Use our suggestions as guides and be creative to adjust to your liking. You don't want to be thinking about our specific instructions when you go down on your lover(s), so feel free to practice in the air or on a carrot while you read so that you can relax and revel in the moment when you eventually get down to business.

Sensual Swipe

Make them crave your touch long after you're gone by exciting one of their hottest spots with your most sensual muscle: your tongue.

Play by play:

▶ Have your lover sit up against the headboard, and kneel between their bent legs.

▶ Wrap both hands around the base of the shaft and lower your moist lips over the head as you suck with shallow strokes, allowing the speed and pressure to increase gradually with each movement.

▶ As tension continues to build, stick your tongue out against the underside of the head and sweep it back and forth over the frenulum at the base of the head. Press with the middle of your tongue as you swipe from side to side like a windshield wiper.

▶ Find a comfortable rhythm and pace and rock your head from side to side to smooth out the movements.

Tantalizing Tip: Lube up your hands before wrapping them around the base of the shaft so you can stroke the lower half while performing the Sensual Swipe.

Tight Tunnel

Use powerful suction to draw their sexual energy to the tip of the penis with your moist lips, and then tease and tantalize as you release your lips on the way back down. Keep them on their toes (and make them curl!) by alternating between intense and tender sensations.

Play by play:

▸ Take some time to arouse their interest with a gentle face caress. Kiss, fondle, and stroke with soft touch, working your way around their jawline, eyebrows, neck, and lips.

▸ As your connection deepens, swipe your cheeks and lips over their chest, working your way down to their abdomen. Roll your tongue around the area and trace the outline of their shaft against their skin.

▸ Moisten your lips and lower them down the shaft as far as you can go without clamping, sucking, or applying pressure.

▸ When you reach your desired depth, seal your lips around the shaft and suck toward the tip with intensity and purpose.

▸ When you reach the top, release your lips and rest them against the head as you twirl your tongue around playfully.

▸ Lower your moist lips back down while breathing out gently, *without* suction or pressure.

▸ Continue to suck upward with all your might and cradle them gently on the way back down.

▸ You can begin with slow, shallow movements and increase the speed and depth with each stroke.

Tantalizing Tip: As their arousal builds and you feel them pulsing or pushing their hips against you, increase the intensity: suck upward several times with all your might, lowering your lips quickly to the base in between each suck. After three tight sucks, slowly and purposefully lower your lips while exhaling and then return to the three powerful sucking motions.

Tongue Cradle

Create a cradle that doubles as a suction cup around the sensitive underside using the wide surface of your tongue to slurp, slide, and suck.

Play by Play:

- Drop to your knees at your lover's feet while they stand against a wall. Use pillows or other soft objects as padding to ensure that you are comfortable.

- Spend a few minutes wandering and exploring between their legs with your lips, tongue, and cheeks, paying extra attention to the inner thighs and stroking their knees and calves with both of your hands.

- Allow your cheeks to brush against their shaft, and lick all around the perineum and balls as you inhale deeply to convey your admiration and pleasure.

- Soak your hands in lube, and when you're both ready, wrap all ten fingers around the base of their shaft to create a tight, wet seal. You can hold your hands still, pulse around the base, swirl around without stroking, or slide up and down the lower third with subtle but deliberate movements.

- Breathe all over the upper half of the shaft and head, teasing with your tongue and lips. After a minute, wrap your wet lips around the upper half and suck while sticking your tongue out. Press your tongue firmly into the underside, allowing it to wrap around and cradle the sides and bottom as you suck with fervor.

- Allow your lips and tongue to work in concert with your hands, and try to create suction with your tongue as opposed to your lips as you envelope the underside with your warm, wet tongue.

Tantalizing Tip: Practice this move on a finger to get a feel for the cradling sensation with your tongue. You may opt to start by rolling your tongue into a tube and wrapping it around your finger before you close your lips. If you cannot roll your tongue into a tube, simply suck on your finger while you press your tongue against the underside; it will likely wrap around your finger naturally as you press and slide.

Hot Damn!

If you like it wet, deep, and tight, the Hot Damn! will be right up your alley. Blend your hands and mouth together to create a seamless tunnel of tight suction.

Play by Play:

▶ Slather your hands in lubricant and place them in prayer position. Push them together to feel the suction you can create with a little lube and pressure.

▶ Place your prayer-position hands in front of your mouth to extend its length (with your thumbs against your lips).

▶ Lower your hands over the head, leading with your pinkie fingers. As you slide down the shaft, squeeze gently with your hands and follow with your mouth, so that your hands and mouth move as one fluid unit.

▶ Move slowly up and down the shaft at first, and increase your speed and pressure as their arousal escalates.

Tantalizing Tip: Your hands will be the first contact point against their sensitive head, but if you want your hands to feel like a true extension of your mouth, "trick" the penis by warming up your hands and breathing heavily as you approach. As they sense your breath, they'll likely anticipate that your mouth will follow.

The Ultimate Three-Way

Take their pleasure to new heights as you simultaneously stimulate the penis, balls, and inner B-spot using your hands, lips, and tongue. As you activate the genital sensory cortex, you will encourage the pleasure and orgasmic response to spread throughout the body.

Play by play:

▸ Trace three lubed-up fingers in a figure-eight formation over their perineum with firm pressure. Work your way up to their balls and cup them in your wet hand, tugging down on them very gently.

▸ Use your other hand to stroke the shaft with lots of lube, and add a firm squeeze or pulse each time you reach the base.

▸ At the same time, suck on the sensitive head while flicking your tongue against the frenulum with every stroke.

▸ This one requires a bit of coordination, so don't get hung up on the specifics of the technique itself; simply stroke, suck, and touch in multiple areas to activate multiple nerve pathways and overwhelm their body with pleasure.

A note on nerves and sex: While the brain is considered the most powerful sex organ and the skin is considered the largest, nerves transmit the signals and impulses to help you recognize, interpret, and enjoy pleasure. Nerves throughout the entire body generate sexual and erotic sensations, and different nerve pathways transmit information from various parts of the genital region. The **pelvic nerve** is believed to convey signals from the vagina, cervix, rectum, and bladder, and **the vagus**

nerve is believed to communicate information from the cervix, uterus, and vagina. **The hypogastric nerve** transmits information from the uterus, cervix, and prostate, and the **pudendal nerve** carries data from the clitoris, penis, and scrotum. As you simultaneously stimulate different areas, you signal pleasure via multiple pathways, which might explain why some orgasms feel more full-bodied.

The Swallower

Lengthen your throat and suck with greater intensity as you tighten your grip and pulse with your hands around the head, shaft, and base.

Play by play:

▶ You can try almost any technique in almost any position, but if you want to get creative, try this one in the Great Gorge(ous) position (see Oral Sex Positions in the next chapter). Lie on your back with your head hanging off the side of the bed. Some people report that this position elongates the mouth and throat, allowing you to slide a little deeper. Your lover stands on the floor next to you, and you can place your hands on their hips to control the depth of penetration.

▶ Suck them into your mouth, and as you do this, be sure you are taken care of too. You can reach down and touch yourself, wear a vibrating toy, or have them bend over and lick, suck, and kiss you between your legs.

▶ As your arousal builds, tighten the grip with your lips and swallow deeply as you suck. You can swallow over the head or against the frenulum to create tension and pulsations as you suck. Or you can lower your lips to the base and swallow deeply several times to allow your muscles to contract around your lover at your maximum desired depth.

▶ Alternate between sucking from base to tip and performing exaggerated swallows in between each sucking stroke.

Tantalizing Tip: If you find yourself gagging on their phallus, you have several options:

▶ If you don't mind the sensation of gagging, lean in and indulge. There is no reason to be self-conscious, as many folks report being turned on by gagging sights and sounds.

▶ If you aren't into gagging, simply adjust your depth and use your wet hands as an extension of your mouth to go a little deeper.

▶ Do more for yourself! When you're turned on, you may find that your gagging reflex becomes less sensitive and your response subsides.

Oral Threesome

Threesomes are among the most common of fantasies for people of all genders. But oftentimes the thought and imagination associated with a fantasy make it hotter than reality itself. The oral threesome allows you to explore this fantasy and take it to the next level.

Play by Play:

▶ Blindfold your lover so that they can focus on your touch and the sound of your voice without any visual distractions.

▶ Explore their entire body using as many points of contact as possible. Kiss their neck while you fondle a nipple with one hand and stroke between their thighs with the other. Taste their hips and abdomen with your tongue and mouth while you caress their balls and trace your palm over their shaft to arouse their interest. Sit on their chest with your butt in their face as you bend over and taste their balls, stroke their shaft, and play with their perineum. Overwhelm them with physical touch across the entire body before you suck them into your mouth.

▶ Enhance the threesome fantasy with dirty talk. *Do you love that? Do you like two of us working over you at once? You deserve more than two hands on your hot body.*

▶ Dance your tongue around their shaft while you "lick" around the head with a wet (lubed-up) finger. Add another finger into the mix so it feels as though they're being overtaken by three tongues.

▶ Suck their head into your mouth while two wet fingers simulate multiple tongues over the shaft and balls. Continue to weave the fantasy by stroking your lover's ego: *Of course I want to share you. I want everyone to know just how good you are. I want them to know how lucky I am.*

▶ Throughout the experience, try to maintain at least three points of contact, and alternate between your lips, tongue, fingers, palms, cheeks, and any other body parts you can throw into the mix so that your partner becomes engulfed in the physical sensations. The sensory deprivation of a blindfold will not only sharpen their other senses, but create a sense of delightful confusion as you overwhelm their body with unpredictable touch.

If threesomes and/or multiple partners are not a part of your sexual agreement, be sure to debrief after you indulge in this fantasy. Ask for and provide reassurance to reinforce the fact that enjoying and indulging in a fantasy need not lead to pursuing the fantasy in real life.

Remember that ongoing communication is of paramount importance to any sexual experience—especially if you are trying something new—so be sure to solicit and share feedback. A gentle tap of the hand, an animalistic groan, and an exaggerated exhale can go a long way to put you both at ease and start important and fruitful conversations.

The Unpredictable Lover

Alternate between deep, powerful sucking and shallow, tender strokes to keep your lover guessing as you tantalize the entire length of their phallus.

Play by Play:

- ▸ Tease your lover throughout the day: flash them as you walk past them working at their computer; send them raunchy song lyrics; text them a naughty close-up so they have to decipher the image; slip them the tongue when you kiss goodbye in the morning; brush against them under the table at dinner; tell them about a saucy dream you had and embellish the details to include them or one of their fantasies.

- ▸ When you're finally alone and have time to connect, kiss them passionately and then pull back to touch their skin flirtatiously with your fingertips.

- ▸ Look up at them and ask them if they want you to wrap your lips around them.

▶ When you are both in the mood, lower yourself to their waist and slide your lips up and down the shaft as though you are running them along the edge of a harmonica—but wetter. Moan so they feel your vibrations and touch yourself so that the blood rushes to your hottest spots too.

▶ When it comes time to suck it right into your mouth, alternate between deep and shallow sucks: lower your lips to the base (you can always use a wet hand as a smooth extension of your mouth) and suck at least three times, squeezing tightly with every suck; then roll your lips up to the head and suck on the head, twirling your tongue around the ridge for three sensuous sucks.

▶ Continue to alternate between deep and shallow sucks, increasing the intensity as you feel the blood engorging the shaft and head. Use the shallow sucks to take a break, and feel free to use your hands to replace your mouth at any point in time.

▶ When you feel a pulsing sensation rushing through the shaft, focus on deep sucks (or pulses with your wet hands) and pick up the pace to one to two sucks per second.

Tantalizing Tip: Try this in multiple positions to discover how your pleasure and comfort, as well as your lover's reactions, change with each new angle.

The Pout

Pout like a supermodel to allow your warm, textured inner cheeks to provide extra friction as you slide and suck from base to tip. Positioning yourself at your lover's side will allow you to create extra friction and heat against the sensitive frenulum and the responsive dorsal vein.

Play by Play:

▶ Kneel at your lover's side so they get a profile view of your body at their waist.

▶ Press your tongue flat against the bottom of your mouth to cover your bottom teeth before lowering your mouth over their head and shaft.

▶ Suck your cheeks in like a supermodel posing with their pout, and allow them to collapse to create a tighter grip.

▶ Exaggerate the sucking-in sensation with your cheeks as you allow them to envelop the entire length of your lover's phallus.

▶ If you need a break as you suck, pop off the top of the head with a wet sucking sensation. Hold their shaft in your hands like an old-fashioned joystick as you look your lover in the eyes to wield your power.

Tantalizing Tip: Get an even tighter grip and give your facial muscles a break by squeezing your cheeks together with your fingers to compress your pout.

The Claudia

Claudia is a physical therapist, masseuse, and the ultimate seductress, and couples come from all corners of the globe to visit her in Mexico, because she creates an experience unlike any other. Using touch techniques that engage the entire body and build a crescendo of desire and tension over the course of several hours, Claudia takes full-body pleasure to a whole new level.

This technique refers specifically to a hand-job approach that has blown thousands of minds. We call it the **hand job to end all blow jobs**. It is that good.

But despite the fact that we've named this technique after Claudia, she isn't a one-trick pony. Her approach isn't just about technique. It is about physical sensuality, connection, energy, and anticipation. As she strokes your bodies (and teaches you to do the same, drawing your partner into the mix), she uses a wide array of techniques that align with her mood and her natural inclinations. It's not memorized or choreographed—it is a genuine experience that culminates in multiple and/or full-body orgasms for those lucky enough to get lost in the process.

Most penises say they found the experience overwhelming—euphoric, even. And when Claudia uses this technique at the end, almost all report that they did not believe that she was only using her hands (they are blindfolded). They assumed that their partner was sucking them off or riding them (Claudia only works with couples) but she really is using nothing but her hands—and twice as much lube as you have ever used.

Of course, the euphoric and orgasmic response isn't a matter of the technique and lube alone. Claudia takes a full hour to touch, caress, and titillate your entire body first (along with your partner). It is the process culminating in this move that makes it so memorable and moving. This, of course, serves as a reminder that the techniques and tips pale in comparison to the buildup and the mood you set. And if you've come this far, we know you already recognize that foreplay begins long before you ever touch; if you wait until you're naked to get to it, it will not have the same impact.

But back to The Claudia—this one is simple.

Play by play:

▸ Take your time to explore the entire body. Can you draw the physical exploration out to twenty minutes? How about forty? The more anticipation you build, the more powerful the orgasmic eruption will be when you finally draw it out.

▶ When the time comes to stroke the penis off, use two hands with your fingers interlaced.

▶ Use twice as much lube as you think you need, and then you can use even more pressure.

▶ Stroke from base to tip with a little extra pressure at the base (along the penis's orgasmic platform).

Tantalizing Tip: Twist your hands over the head with every stroke. Allow your hands to twirl around in a rhythmic fashion as you squeeze at the base and swirl at the head, increasing the speed and pressure with every stroke.

Climb into the Cave!

Whether you are stroking with both hands, doing your best version of The Claudia, or flipping your hand upside down (starting in a thumbs-down position) to create a unique sensation while you twist over the head, we implore you to climb into the cave and play with the balls if your flexibility, anatomy, and positioning allow. Here are some possible approaches to consider.

Play by play:

▶ Trace your wet fingers all around the scrotal sac with a barely there touch while you are making out.

▶ Slide your palm along the back of the balls while you press them into your own face, and draw a big slow W over the front side.

▶ Gently suck only on the skin of the scrotal sac, adding a few drops of lube to tone down the suction.

▸ As your lover becomes aroused, you will likely observe that the scrotal sac tightens; at this point, gently suck a whole ball (or two!) into your mouth and swirl your tongue all around.

▸ Paint figure-eight patterns over the scrotal sac with your tongue or a soft makeup brush covered in lubricant.

▸ Cup the balls with one hand and gently tug them downward as you suck the penis from base to tip; press the balls up slightly as you slide your mouth back down to the base of the penis.

▸ Slather lube all over the balls and rub your face in it as you inhale and exhale with rapture and/or devotion.

▸ Roll a bullet vibe or a soft flat vibrator all around the balls with a few drops of lube.

▸ Suck on the balls while you stroke the phallus.

▸ Roll the backs of your fingernails all around as you look them in the eye. Be sure to use your lubricant!

▸ Lightly brush the scrotal sac with your fingertips or nails.

▸ Use light pinches with your index finger and thumb or between your index finger and middle finger to grab the skin of the scrotal sac.

▸ While sucking, use the tips of your fingers to tickle the perineum and the scrotal sac for an interesting sensation.

The Mind-Blower

This finishing move builds upon The Claudia, bringing the warmth and intimacy of your mouth into the mix to create more tension and suction as you stroke your lover into sexual oblivion.

Play by Play:

▸ Pick a position that doesn't require that you hold yourself upright with your core muscles. You will not have access to your hands, as they will be wrapped around the shaft the entire time, so find a position in which you can lean on your elbows comfortably. Kneeling on the floor at the side of the bed or lying on your side in a facing-spoons position might be most comfortable.

▸ Play with your lover in any way that appeals to you: slather your body in oil and rub yourself all over them from head to toe, or tie their hands behind their back and tease them with just your tongue until they are begging you to take them in your mouth.

▸ Build arousal and pleasure slowly: paint lube over their shaft with a soft makeup brush and then rub your cheeks against them to build warmth. Lick from base to tip and then run your nose down the wet paths you've created around the entire circumference. Suck them into your mouth, inching your way down slowly and sucking up quickly. Pop off the top like you are sucking on the most delicious lollipop you've ever tasted.

▸ When you can feel them throbbing with delight, take them over the edge by attaching your hands to your mouth to create a long, warm, wet tunnel of suction. Use both hands and interlace your fingers (as you would in The Claudia), using a generous serving of lube and more pressure than you are accustomed to—especially over the lower third of the shaft. Most of us do not use enough pressure when sucking and stroking because we don't use enough lube; saliva is lovely, but it tends to dry out more quickly and doesn't allow you to squeeze, twist, and slide with the same dexterity as a few drops of lube. And as you blend your saliva with a little lube, you will create a slippery concoction that will make every touch and movement more gratifying and delightful.

▶ Pick up the pace as you stroke and suck, and try to ensure that your hands remain in contact with your mouth so it feels like a never-ending vacuum of wet suction and pressure.

Yes. No. Maybe.

Up your game by making small movements that will keep them guessing and help you to relax into the moment.

Play by Play:

▶ Greet your lover in an unexpected place (e.g., their home office or the kitchen) in a partial state of undress. You might wear your regular top, but remove your bra or wear something short with no underwear. Alternatively, you might greet them topless but wearing your favorite jeans. Regardless of gender, visual seduction can enhance any sexual interaction—especially if *you* take pride and pleasure in your body.

▶ Have your lover sit on the counter or on a chair as you climb between their legs.

▶ Breathe loudly, exhaling through your mouth, and rub your face in their crotch. Nod your head up and down as though you are nodding *yes*, and back and forth as though you are shaking your head *no*. Allow your ears, hair, nose, and cheeks to rub against them through their clothing.

▶ Look up at them and unbutton, unzip, or pull their pants

or skirt out of the way. Trace your hands around their head and shaft. Use one hand to press a vibrator (or three fingers) against their perineum and the other to press on their pucker firmly, but without penetration.

▸ Suck them into your mouth and find a slow rhythm that works for you. When you are ready, nod your head as though you're saying yes and continue to suck up and down. If you don't want to go deep, use your wet hand as an extension of your mouth.

▸ Alternate between a few strokes nodding *yes* and a few strokes shaking your head *no* to find a natural pace and groove.

▸ You can nod as you stroke downward or upward, or you can only nod when you arrive at their swollen head, while you stick your tongue out to sweep against the underside where the head and shaft meet.

▸ Do what feels more comfortable and move in a way that feels natural. You might suck with fervent delight for a few strokes and then suck as you nod back and forth over the head, continuing to alternate between the two. Or you might suck as deep as possible and nod your head up and down as you swallow at the very bottom, or from side to side as you exhale and allow yourself to gag gently.

Tantalizing Tip: Try this one in the sixty-nine position so you can get yours too!

The Facial
You do not need to come on your lover's face to enjoy a sexual facial. You can also use your face to rile your lover into a frenzy as they watch you rubbing yourself with passion against their most sensitive spots.

Play by Play:

▶ Position yourself between your lover's legs so that they have a full view of your face.

▶ Look up into their eyes as you unhurriedly draw their head into your mouth and press it into your cheeks, so that they can see its outline poking through.

▶ Close your lips as you pop it back out and run your lips over the tip.

▶ Use a sloppy tongue to soak the entire length of their phallus (and balls) before rubbing your face all over the area. Get your cheeks wet, close your eyes, and inhale deeply to convey your delight.

▶ Suck them into your mouth again, working from base to tip for a few strokes, and then pop the head through your lips so you can get your face deep into the area. Rub all over with your cheeks, chin, and lips, allowing your face to get wet and breathing it all in.

▶ Talk dirty, begging your lover to come all over you. (You can start dropping less explicit hints earlier in the day. *I want to watch you finish later.*) Ask for it wherever you want it—on your face, your chest, your stomach, your legs, your back, or in your mouth.

▶ Use your hands to guide the direction and "landing zone" if and when you opt to suck them off to orgasm/ ejaculation.

Coming on your partner's face is neither inherently degrading nor universally desired. It is a top fantasy for some of us, and others have no interest in it, despite its common depiction as the norm in porn. Some embrace the consensual degradation (power play), while others see it as an act of validation. It's important to remember that no consensual sex act is inherently *anything*. If you are into facials, it's not a sign that you're empowered, and it's not a sign that you are subjugated. If you're into submission, it might be because you want to relinquish the powerful roles you play in real life, or it might simply be because it feels physically and emotionally good to play a sub. You are the only one who can determine why you enjoy a specific act and you do not owe anyone an explanation. In fact, you may not even want to explore why you want what you want, and that's okay too. The bottom line: you do you.

Pleasure Twist

The nerve-rich head of the penis is sensitive to touch, pressure, temperature, texture, and moisture. Roll your tongue over this region as you suck to spark new sensations in this highly erogenous area.

Play by Play:

▶ Lie side by side on the bed and wrap one hand around the base of your lover's shaft.

▶ Resist the urge to suck them into your mouth right away. Instead, flutter your tongue along their abdomen, allowing it to lick the shaft if it gets in the way.

▶ Run your tongue along the raphe and then curl your lips into a little circle to blow cool air over your wet path. The raphe is the dividing line that stretches from the anus over the center of their perineum to the balls and all the way up to the tip of the penis.

▶ Swipe your tongue around the head and shaft, working your way up and down as though your tongue is dancing on a pole.

▶ When you're ready, close your lips and suck away at a rhythmic pace while your tongue continues to dance around the pole.

▶ As you suck toward the top of the shaft, feel the frenulum between your lips, and sweep your tongue over it in a J shape with firm pressure. You might find that a little turn of your head helps to facilitate the simultaneous sucking and flicking.

▶ As you suck, reach down between their legs and use all five fingers (with lube) to stroke in an oval shape over the million-dollar point.

▶ If you need a break from all the action, douse your hands in lube, stroke with all ten fingers interlaced, and bury your head in their body as you catch your breath.

Tantalizing Tip: As an alternative to sweeping your tongue over the frenulum, alternate between sucking with your tongue pressed against the underside of the head for a few strokes and sliding (the underside of) your tongue onto the upper side of the head. Try it on your finger first: suck with your tongue underneath your finger and then slide your tongue over the top. It sounds complicated, but it should flow smoothly if you practice on your finger first to develop the muscle memory.

Tightest Hold

This powerful blow job technique offers the tightest squeeze possible as you clench your lover's phallus between your teeth, but use the soft padding of your lips and tongue to ensure it is a smooth, pain-free ride—unless you are into pain, which is okay too.

Play by play:

▸ Suck with all your might while creating a tight clamp using the pressure of your teeth. Cover your lower teeth with your tongue and wrap your upper lip around your upper row of teeth to create a tight seal while you suck.

▸ Use a little lube on your upper lip. Increase the pressure at the base while easing up a little as you approach the head.

▸ This is a tiring technique, and you likely cannot keep it up for minutes at a time, so be sure to use a few of the seduction and erotic touch techniques we've already discussed to amplify arousal across their body before trying the Tightest Hold.

Tantalizing Tip: Let your slurps, sucks, and other natural sex sounds run amok! Sex is supposed to be a sensual experience, and sound is an often-undervalued erotic sense. So do not hold back. Breathe deeply and let your naughty noises come out to play!

The Game Changer

If you want to ensure mutual enjoyment in any sexual experience, you need to be comfortable and confident. When it comes to blow jobs, it's not uncommon for folks of all genders to express discomfort with deep throating and exhaustion with the whole process itself. As hot as blow jobs may be, sucking, stroking, and bobbing up and down can tire out the muscles in your face, jaw, neck, and mouth. Enter The Game Changer. This simple approach to blow jobs can alleviate the muscular pressure while allowing you to maintain the right type of pressure around the base, shaft, and head of your favorite phallus.

Play by play:

▶ Warm your lover up with some tongue-only action to tease them to attention: trace the outline around their abs, lick a line from base to tip of their phallus, draw wide figure-eight symbols over the balls, and press your tongue flat against the head.

▶ Gradually lower your wet lips over the head and release some warm air without sealing your lips. Repeat several times until they start "bouncing" at you or trying to press into your lips.

▶ As you pick up the pace, slide up and down, experiment with tongue twirling, play with small twists over the head, or suck their balls right into your mouth until the entire head and shaft are swelling and pulsing with desire.

▶ As arousal is about to peak, pull out The Game Changer: wrap your lips around and suck with all your might, but **use your fingers to create the pressure and grip**. Place your index finger above your upper lip and your thumb under your lower lip and pinch them together. Your face and jaw can relax as you keep your lips wrapped around your lover, but allow your fingers to squeeze them together and do the real work.

▶ You will likely find that you can maintain pressure and suction for a longer period of time with the help of your fingers, and your lover will still benefit from the physical sensations, visual appeal, and psychological excitement of your wet, willing mouth around their phallus.

Tantalizing Tip: Change the position of your lips and fingers to create new sensations, and your partner will benefit from the excitement of unpredictability. You can squeeze your lips around the top and bottom of the penis or rotate your fingers to squeeze your lips together and create more friction from the sides. Alternatively, change it up and squeeze only at the base or only as you pass over the corona (the bulging ridge at the bottom of the head).

Slow Job

This sensuous blow job move is designed to make your lover's body writhe with pleasure by using moderate deprivation to build an orgasm of dramatic and unrivaled magnitude.

Play by play:

▸ Find your way to your lover's feet, and if you are both open to it, set the mood with a sensual foot massage. Slide your thumbs in circular motions against the soles of their feet using a massage oil or lotion. Pet their upper feet with wide, flat palms and medium pressure. Roll each toe between your index finger and thumb. Rub the entire length of their feet between your two hands as though you are warming them up.

▸ Work your way up to their calves, wrapping your entire hands around them and rotating smoothly, with each hand turning in the opposite direction (as though you are gently wringing out laundry).

▸ When you arrive at their thighs, continue to sweep your palms over them from side to side, and add kisses and the twirl of your tongue as you approach their groin.

▸ Trace your tongue around the outline of their phallus. Nibble playfully on it with no teeth. Stick your lips out and run them along its length. Swirl your tongue around the head as you tease with your warm breath and wet mouth.

▶ When you're ready to swallow them into your mouth, move slowly—millimeter by millimeter. Rest your lips on the tip to build anticipation. Open s-l-o-w-l-y and take at least one full minute to glide your lips over the head, past the corona, down the shaft, all the way to the base.

▶ Take a few deep breaths at the base—and remember that you can always use your hands covered in lube as an extension of your mouth, so there is no pressure to deep-throat with your mouth alone.

▶ Slide back up almost as slowly as you worked your way down.

▶ Continue for several full-length strokes, moving at this unnaturally slow pace until the rhythm begins to feel natural.

▶ You can maintain this slow pace throughout the entire sexual experience or opt to use it as part of your seduction routine before moving on to more robust activities. You may also use it to break up your sex play or prolong the experience through the practice of edging.

The more slowly you move, the more likely you will be to take note of every texture, curve, angle, sound, and feeling. You will likely feel as though their phallus is *too big*—as though it is exploding in your mouth with every tiny movement. You may also have difficulty breathing with your mouth full, so don't be afraid to come up for air and take a moment for yourself. Hold their shaft in your hands as you look them in the eye and savor every slow breath.

Oftentimes, we associate orgasm with rapid, rhythmic stroking and sucking (one to two strokes per second), but you can also induce orgasmic contractions and sexual climax with slow, purposeful touch. You may even find that the response is more full-bodied as you draw awareness away from the genitals themselves and tap into the full potential of your breath and the expanse of your skin from the top of your scalp to the tips of your toes.

A note on edging: Edging often refers to bringing yourself right to the brink of orgasm several times without allowing yourself to go over the edge.

Most people learn and practice edging on their own before involving a partner. For example, you might rile yourself up with your hands or toys, but stop or slow down as soon as you feel as though you're about to climax. Breathe deeply as you retreat to a less stimulating technique or area until the urge to orgasm subsides. You can repeat this process several times. Most people want to maintain sexual arousal throughout the process, as opposed to allowing sexual desire to subside altogether. As you experiment with edging, pay attention to how you feel in your body—you might feel greater intensity in your groin, but many people report feeling more full-body pleasure when they prolong the sexual experience.

Couples often experiment with edging to delay and/or intensify orgasm or to maintain a heightened state of pleasure for an extended period of time. You might pleasure your partner until they give you a sign that orgasm is about to happen; at this point, you can stop, slow down, or move to a different type of stimulation that is less likely to lead to orgasm. Once they've calmed down, you can bring them back up to the brink of orgasm and repeat several times. When they eventually reach orgasm, they might feel that it is more powerful—the contractions may be stronger and more numerous, the pleasure might be deeper, it might last longer, and they may feel a wave of pleasure over their entire body.

Some people enjoy hierarchical edging: think about arousal on a numerical scale, with zero representing no arousal and ten representing orgasm. Touch yourself (or your partner) until your arousal reaches a level six and then allow the pleasure to subside to a four. Rile yourself up again until you are a seven and then drop to a four. Follow this pattern with an eight and then a nine until you are ready to go over the edge. Of course, you cannot perfectly assess arousal levels, and it doesn't have to be an incremental climb—experiment with different levels and approaches to see what works for you.

In a kinky context, you might experiment with edging as part of orgasm control or denial. For example, you might take your partner to the brink of orgasm and then exercise your power or control to deny them orgasm (with consent). This can heighten feelings of both dominance and submission, as well as allow you to play with elements of objectification, surrender, and torture.

Irrumatio

Part of the allure and intoxication of giving head involves the interplay of both dominance and submission in both the giver and receiver roles. When you take your lover into your mouth, you can choose to subjugate yourself physically (e.g., at their feet) and emotionally (e.g., at their service), but you can also play a dominant role with your lover's most tender tendril against your sharp teeth. When receiving oral pleasure, you place yourself at their mercy, while simultaneously maintaining some control over their airway with your phallus inches away from their throat.

Most blow jobs focus on the act of *fellatio*, in which the giver maintains primary control of the movements, speed, suction, depth, and technique. You may, however, also want to experiment with *irrumatio*, in which the penis takes over and glides into its partner's mouth as it wishes.

With all sexual interactions, discuss your desires and boundaries ahead of time, and since a safe word will not suffice with your mouth full, devise a **safe signal** in advance. For example, you might snap your fingers or raise your hands to indicate that you are feeling uncomfortable and want to stop. **Safe words** and **safe signals** are coded responses that allow you to clearly and immediately communicate your limits and needs. "Stop" may not suffice if it is a part of your sexual fantasy or role-play, and no safe word will work if your speech is inhibited by a gag or a penis in your mouth.

You may also want to develop a nonverbal communication code to avoid having to interrupt a sexual interaction to have a long-form conversation. For example, you can hold up your fingers to indicate how much more pressure or penetration you desire, ranging from zero to five, where zero indicates that you cannot take any more and five indicates that your lover should ramp it up.

Safe words and signals should be clearly defined, and if you want to stop or have changed your mind about any activity, you shouldn't hesitate to use yours with the expectation that your partner will respond immediately.

Play by play:

▶ Kiss, caress, hug, snuggle, and get close to one another so that you're feeling relaxed and building desire. Allow your bodies to intertwine as you reap the benefits of physical touch from head to toe. Don't feel the need to reach down between one another's legs right away. Allow the excitement to build and enjoy the rush of oxytocin, which not only has the potential to deepen bonding, but also to promote trust.

▸ Have your lover go down on you first or pleasure you in a way that puts you at ease before you suck them into your mouth.

▸ Take a minute to lick, suck, breathe, and swirl around their shaft, and when you're ready, let them know that they can begin to slide in and out of your mouth at their leisure. You may want to wrap your hand (covered in lube) around the base of their shaft to limit the depth of penetration.

▸ Your lover can adjust the speed, angle, and rhythm of thrusting, being mindful of your reactions; this means that they'll need to keep their eyes open to watch for your signal(s). We suggest that they start more slowly and gently and increase the speed and depth of penetration as your arousal climbs. Your lover may wish to place their hands on the back of your head (if you're comfortable with it).

▸ Remember that you will both derive greater pleasure from the experience if you check in with one another often.

The Extenderator

Extend your stroke to include the inner penis by coordinating your movements along the outer penis with the pressure you apply to the inner penis.

Play by play:

▸ Kneel between your lover's legs and stroke their inner thighs as you taste their balls and roll your tongue around the base of the shaft.

▸ Work them up using any of the techniques you love and then seal your wet lips around the shaft to suck from base to tip. You can cover your teeth with your lips to get a tighter grip or press a vibrator against your cheek to allow the reverberations to punctuate every stroke.

▸ As you suck, press your index, middle, and ring fingers along the perineum right behind the balls. Be sure to add lube.

▸ As you lower your lips down to the base, press your warm, lubricated fingers against their perineum and stroke backward toward the butt; this is a tiny movement—perhaps a half-inch stroke.

▸ As you suck back up toward the top, slide your fingers forward toward the balls with firm pressure.

▸ Envision your fingers as an extension of your mouth and the perineum an extension of the penis. Stroke and suck in rhythm so that your fingers move back (toward the butt) as your lips move down toward the base and your fingers move forward toward the balls as you suck toward the tip of the penis.

▸ Do not get hung up on the coordination. Simply allow your fingers to follow the movement and rhythm of your lips, which in turn are guided by the rhythm of your lover's hips.

Tantalizing Tip: If coordinating movements between your mouth and hands feels unnatural or distracts you from the pleasure of the experience, forget about your finger and simply press a powerful vibrating toy against the perineum.

Prostate Play

To excite and stimulate the prostate externally, apply pressure or vibrations along the perineum toward the back (near the anus). The sling of muscles that supports this area is quite thick, so light pressure will stimulate nerve endings in a pleasurable way (perfect for inciting interest during the early stages of seduction), but if you want to specifically fire up the prostate, you will need to apply pressure. Curl your fingers in either direction just in front of the pucker, or pulse with a flat palm against the full length of the perineum during oral, manual, or any other type of sex.

Should you find that your lover enjoys external prostate play, you may also want to consider internal stimulation (sometimes referred to as *milking*). Because the prostate sits against the rectal wall, you can curl a finger or toy into the anus to tease, please, and massage this sensitive gland. You might curl your fingers up toward the stomach and press against the upper wall to arouse the swollen gland in a come-hither motion. Alternatively, you can slide a finger back and forth from left to right with a tiny movement in a cupping motion.

If you are stroking the penis, you might want to throb a finger against the prostate in rhythm with your strokes, or you can use a toy like the **Aneros Progasm Jr.** or the **Aneros Helix Syn**—both allow for self-pleasure and provide stimulation internally against the prostate and externally along the perineum and beyond. They are considered hands-free toys and respond to even tiny contractions, so you will have your hands free to wander over their body. Should you prefer a vibrating massager, the **Aneros Vice** offers a range of vibrations from the subtle to the intense that can be felt beyond the prostate in the anal canal and full pelvic region.

Note on prostate orgasms: Brain scan research suggests that there may be different *types* of orgasm and the site of stimulation may play a role in how we experience pleasure. Prostate orgasms, for example, are often described as full-body experiences, and many folks with penises report that prostate massage can produce overwhelming pleasure, release, and contractions without ever touching the penis. Of course, you don't need to check specific *types* of orgasm off your sexual bucket list. It can be difficult, if not impossible, to perfectly differentiate between various pathways to orgasm, so rather than worrying about the *type* of orgasm, focus on the experience itself. You will be a far more appealing lover if you zone in on the pleasure and connection as opposed to an expected goal or outcome.

Notes on Anal Penetration

Whether you are putting a toy, a finger, a penis, or another body part in your butt, remember that foreplay is your friend. Just as you wouldn't walk in the door and put your finger in your partner's mouth (or vagina), the butt requires some pre-lovin' before it will invite you in to play. Consider the following before experimenting with anal play:

Use lube. Many people opt for silicone-based formulas for anal play, as they tend to be more slippery and longer lasting. Whatever formulation you choose, use twice as much as you think you will need and keep it on hand in case you need more. The anus does not create enough lubrication for penetration, so lube is absolutely necessary. Note: you might notice some fluid secretion during arousal and orgasm, and this may be related to both sweat and the secretion of mucus from the rectum, but it is not generally enough to facilitate pleasurable penetration.

Get to know *your* butt first. You may not be able to look inside, but you can still become best of friends. On the outside, you've got your butt hole (AKA pucker), which tends to be highly responsive to light touch, textures, and temperature. We share some moves to play with your pucker on the next page.

Once you slide inside, you arrive at the sensitive anal canal, and you will feel two ringlike muscles: your anal sphincters (it is fun to say *sphincters* out loud). The external sphincter (located just inside the opening) is controlled by your central nervous system, so you can contract and release it at will. Just beyond the first ring muscle, you will find the internal sphincter, which is controlled by the autonomic nervous system and remains in a state of partial contraction. Just as you cannot fully control your heartbeat or blood pressure, you cannot exercise total control over this involuntary muscle; you can, however, encourage it to release by relaxing, breathing deeply, and indulging in pleasure.

Before you put anything in someone else's butt, please practice penetrating your own butt first to become acquainted with your sphincter friends. Breathe deeply, use lube, get aroused, and slide your finger inside while you contract and release the external sphincter around its tip. Try this a few times until you feel comfortable with the shallow insertion. This could take a few days, a few weeks, or longer. There is no rush.

Once you and the external sphincter become friends, slide just a little deeper and breathe as you become familiar with the internal sphincter. Can you breathe more slowly and deeply to recognize its response? If you are not relaxed, it can be painful, so bear this in mind when you are considering a visit to your lover's butt. Which brings us to the next point . . .

Move slowly and gradually. Anal penetration should not be painful, so move slowly. Start with a small object like your pinkie finger or a narrow toy with a flared base. Gradually increase the depth and size over time.

Only use toys designed specifically for anal play. Never use a small object without a flared base (or stopper) in the anus. Unlike the vagina, which is a defined space ending at the cervix, the anus leads to the rectum and intestines. You do not want to lose a toy up there, so a flared base, ring, or other stopper is a must.

Rile yourself up first. Arousal has a palliative effect on the body. Sensations that are experienced as uncomfortable or even painful in an unaroused state can feel intensely pleasurable as your sexual excitement soars. You might even want to have an orgasm before you consider venturing inside, as the endorphin and oxytocin surge can remain elevated post-orgasm.

Of course, penetration is always optional—for every orifice— so read on to discover techniques and approaches that facilitate backdoor play without ever crossing the internal threshold.

Pucker Stuff: For All Bodies!

The anus is a nerve-ending hotbed, and for many anal sex aficionados, the best anal sex happens on the *outside*. Oftentimes, people will avoid butt stuff, as they believe that it's dirty or they worry that playing on the outside will inevitably lead to penetration, but this need not be the case. You can have smokin'-hot anal sex by playing with the sensitive pucker and its neighbors, the cheeks and crack.

The techniques below are merely guidelines. You don't have to follow each tip sequentially. If you find something that works, stick with it!

▸ Plant featherlight kisses with wet lips all over your lover's butt cheeks.

▸ Add your tongue to your kisses, wiggling it in between their butt cheeks.

▸ Apply your favorite flavored lube and rub it in with two thumbs.

▸ Press your tongue flat again the pucker (bum hole) and curl it upward.

▸ Paint, twirl, and lick around your lover's pucker teasingly.

▸ Swivel your tongue around in a figure-eight shape over their perineum and bum hole.

▸ Use two hands to spread your lover's butt cheeks, and press your lips around the pucker while twirling your tongue in circular motions.

▸ Change directions with your tongue and widen your licks into large ovals. Alternate between wet oval-shaped strokes with a wide, flat tongue and short flicks with just the tip.

▸ When you are both feeling ready and relaxed, stick out your tongue and glide the tip in and out of the pucker. Your lover will need to relax to allow your soft tongue to slide in.

▸ Wiggle your tongue up and town, side to side, and in circular motions as you penetrate your lover's warm pucker.

▸ Reach one lubed-up hand around and stroke their cock in rhythm with your sucking and licking.

POSITIONS, PERVERTABLES, PROPS—OH MY!

Oral Sex Positions

We believe that comfort outranks technique when it comes to sex—including oral sex. Oftentimes, we avoid certain sex acts or cut them short because they are uncomfortable or tiring. We may also find that we're distracted and less mindful of pleasure and connection if our muscles are fatigued or we're focused on holding ourselves up. Repositioning is therefore key to mind-blowing oral sex, so we've outlined thirteen oral sex positions to ensure that sex is both pleasurable and cozy.

Each of these oral sex positions offers general recommendations, but you are the expert when it comes to your own body, so it's up to you to experiment and adapt these positions to suit them to your pleasure.

All Fours
This position allows your lover(s) to access you from the front or from the rear and allows you to control the depth and the pressure, since you are on top.

▶ Get on your hands and knees and wait for your partner to position themselves.

▶ Your lover can approach you from behind or slide underneath you while lying on their back.

▶ Modify this position into the All-Fours Stretch—stretch your arms out in front of you (like a cat or dog stretching) and bring your chest down against the mattress to angle your bottom up for improved access. Add a pillow or two beneath your knees for support or if you want an even more dramatic angle.

Indulge Me

This position is perfect for relaxing and taking in the view.

▶ Sit down with your back resting against the wall, headboard, or other flat surface.

▶ With your knees bent, spread your legs wide-open with your feet flat against the floor or bed.

▶ Watch your lover give you pleasure or, to heighten your other senses, use a blindfold!

The Delegator

In this position, you can direct your lover and adjust the pressure, depth, and speed using your hips and/or your hands against the back of their head.

▶ Sit upright in a chair or on the edge of the bed with your legs spread wide.

▶ Place a large pillow underneath your feet as a cushion for their knees or butt, and have them crawl between your legs.

▸ Guide them with your hands on their back or on their head, or use your hips to steer them.

▸ Lift your leg(s) up and wrap them around their neck and shoulders to get closer and provide additional direction using your body, by pulling them in and adjusting the angle.

Superhero

It's a bird, it's a plane, it's, it's . . . it's you flying high on orgasmic air! This position is great for oral and manual sex, regardless of whether you are licking a vulva, an anus, or a penis.

▸ Lie flat on your stomach with your arms stretched out straight and legs spread apart.

▸ Your lover can lie between your legs to access from the rear or they can lie on top of you (with their feet at your head) to use their hands, toys, or mouth.

▸ Change it up with the Reverse Superhero and simply lie on your back with a pillow beneath your hips to angle them up for improved comfort and access.

Flying High

This position allows easy access to your anus, perineum, and lower genitals.

▸ Lie on your back and bend your knees with your legs open wide.

▸ Lift one leg up and place it on your lover's back so that they can climb even deeper between your legs.

Your Royal Highness

Your lover's head and face are now your throne. From this position, you can move up and down as you please according to your desired pressure, depth, rhythm, and speed.

▶ Your lover gets comfortable and lies on their back with pillows underneath their head, neck, and/or shoulders as needed.

▶ Kneel over their head and sit on their face. Be sure they can breathe, and use a safe signal if you are limiting their vocal sounds.

Rise & Shine

Break the routine of having sex in bed. We know it's comfortable, but you can find other comfortable locations throughout your home—and beyond. Breaking the routine of the bedroom (and particularly the bed) can encourage your body to interpret pleasure in new ways, and engaging in new environments can heighten your sexual response to spontaneity. This position also allows you to explore feelings of power and d ominance.

▶ Find a fun spot against a wall and stand straight up with your feet spread hip distance apart.

▶ Your lover gets down at your feet and kneels or crouches as they please you from below.

▶ Stay strong and make sure that you do not get weak in the knees!

Rhythm & Beats

Set the mood with your favorite music playing in the background.

- ▸ Lie on your stomach with your legs hanging off the side of the bed, table, or couch. Spread them open.

- ▸ Your lover kneels or crouches on the floor and licks, kisses, grinds, and moves to the beat of the music. Alternatively, they can lie on top of you to approach from the top.

- ▸ Allow yourself to get lost in the music, movements, and especially, the moment.

The Glee T

Approaching from the side can be a fun and creative approach, as your partner can use their hands on your body and mouth on your genitals, or vice versa.

- ▸ Lie on your back and prop up your hips with a small pillow.

- ▸ Have your lover lie perpendicular to you (so that your bodies form a T) with their head at your crotch.

The High-Riser

If you like real estate, you will love the High-Riser. It has everything you need to have a good time—a phenomenal view, a favorable location, and private access! It's a win-win, as it promotes orgasms for all parties and offers a high return on investment.

- ▸ Lie on your back with a pillow under your head.

- ▸ Your lover straddles your head or chest, facing toward your feet. They bend over and go to town.

- ▸ You can also play with them from behind should the mood strike.

The Acrobat

Throw your legs up and treat yourself to a full-access oral session.

▶ Lie on your back and throw your feet up in the air. Grab hold of your ankles with your hands for support.

▶ Have your lover go down on you, and adjust the angles of your legs to suit your fancy. They can access your butt and genitals from this position, so do not be shy about asking for more, more, and more.

Facing Spoons

This position may be the most comfortable depending on your body types, and remember, comfort makes for hotter sex.

▶ Lie on your sides facing one another and have your lover slide down between your legs.

▶ You can open your legs so that they can slide an arm in between for both comfort and rear access.

The Great Gorge(ous)

Porn depicts deep-throating as the norm, so it's a common fantasy for people of all genders. You or your partner do not have to have a penis to enjoy the thrill and challenge of deep-throating, as a strap-on will also do the trick. This position, also described in the Swallower technique in the previous chapter, allows you to elongate your neck, but it is not a quick fix that will make deep-throating effortless. It takes time, practice, and patience, and you can always use your hands as an extension of your mouth in the meantime (as explained in the Hot Damn and Extenderator techniques).

▶ Lie on your back with your head hanging off the side of the bed.

▶ Have your partner stand in front of you and slide inside your mouth; place your hands on your partner's thighs and brace yourself so that you can control their movements.

▶ Your partner can also bend over and give you a good licking and/or sucking.

SEDUCTION INSTRUCTION

Try some of these positions right now when you are fully clothed. Talk about what works and what doesn't, and see where the discussion and physical experimentation leads.

Seduction and Foreplay Props

Sometimes your bare hands and bare bodies are all you need to pique your partner's interest and seduce them into a sensational sexual experience. Other times, however, props and toys can come in handy, as they add variety, novelty, and unpredictability to sexual interactions. Below, we outline a range of toys you can use to entice your lover(s) and inspire you to try new things—on your own and together. These items are just the beginning, and your options are endless. And remember that you don't have to spend another dollar to enrich your sex life, as you probably own more sex toys than you realize. Be sure to read on to discover what pervertables you have lying around in plain sight.

Vibrators come in a wide variety of sizes, shapes, and textures, and many are designed ergonomically, guided by sexual science. They can be used on the entire body to spread sensations of pleasure across the chest, thighs, perineum, and, of course, the genitals. You can find vibrators that are shaped like penises, as well as a variety of designs that look like common household items (e.g., computer mouse or lipstick) or design pieces you can leave on your mantel or bedside table.

Some of our favorite vibrators include:

Crave Vesper—this beautiful vibrator doubles as jewelry, and its design is subtle and tasteful. Only those in the know will recognize that the art piece hanging from your neck is also a high-end vibrator.

The Hitachi Magic Wand—if you like power, pressure, and coverage, you cannot do better than this gadget. Though the company continues to market it as a personal massager, we all know that its use extends far beyond working the kinks out of your shoulders.

We-Vibe Tango—this is one powerful and versatile bullet vibe. Roll it around on the outside, slide it inside, or press its flat tip against your hottest spots to intensify orgasmic pleasure.

Womanizer Premium—the Womanizer products use pleasure-air technology—tiny bursts of air that create a suction-like sensation over the head of the clit with a round, open tip. Many clients also use it on the nipples and along the labia to stimulate the inner bulbs of the clitoris. Several clients have learned to orgasm for the very first time with the Womanizer products, and the educational staff at Good for Her (Carlyle Jansen's sex-positive shop in Toronto) say it is like having an orgasm again for the very first time. The products come in different models and sizes—we like the Womanizer Premium version because it has an autopilot mode, which offers random patterns of pleasure that add an element of unpredictability.

We-Vibe Sync—designed to be worn during penis-in-vagina intercourse, this toy revolutionized the sex toy industry with its form, function, and app connectivity. The small, flat inner arm vibrates against the G-spot, and the outer arm curves around to vibrate against the hood, shaft, and head of the external clitoris. As you slide your penis or strap-on into the vagina, you benefit from the dual-motor vibrations, which you can program to your liking. The customizable vibrations, app-enabled control, and the option to have the Sync vibe to the beat of your favorite song make this toy highly sought after and unique.

Crave Wink—this one is a beauty, but it is more than just a pretty face. Its silicone and metal composition conduct vibrations with exceptional intensity, making it a standout powerhouse in a pretty, discreet package. If you like marathon sex, this will be your go-to, as it lasts and lasts with a run time of up to five hours. We're exhausted just thinking about it, but we do love a challenge.

Fun Factory Volta—with two vibrating tips, this tulip-like vibe is perfect for the clitoris, nipples, penile frenulum, and any other region that craves deep, rumbly vibrations.

Penis rings are designed to be worn by penises and strap-ons. They trap the blood in the penis to offer the sensation of a harder, fuller erection. Some say penis rings help them to remain erect longer, and some find the pleasure is overwhelming and they reach orgasm more quickly and intensely—luckily, sex isn't something you time.

> Note on erections and timing: you do not get extra points for lasting longer in terms of maintaining an erection. Sexual pleasure doesn't require an erection, and there are a wide range of sexual exploits you can explore with a soft penis, as well as with your hands, mouth, fingers, tongue, toys, and the rest of your body.

Some penis rings are stretchy and others are adjustable in size. Some vibrate and some don't. Some sit at the base of the penis, while others wrap all the way around the base of the penis and the scrotal sac. Two fan favorites include:

We-Vibe Pivot—We do not have penises, but we can attest to the fact that the Pivot works wonders if your partner has a penis, and it can enhance strap-on sex too. This one receives rave reviews from folks of all genders, and its design allows its powerful vibrations to be enjoyed in multiple positions. Regardless of your genital combination, you will find a spot that allows it to vibe just right.

Fun Factory Flame—a more basic, stretchy model without vibrations. Its outer edges provide additional stimulation to the partner during intercourse, and its lower price point makes it a good starter model if you are new to penis rings.

Penis strokers enhance the sensation of stroking the shaft and head of the penis. Some, like the **Tenga Eggs**, are made of elastomer with textured internal details and are designed for single use (although we use them more than once). Others, like the **Hot Octopuss Pulse III Solo**, use oscillations to do the work for you—you do not even have to stroke (but you can if you want to), as the oscillations can produce overpowering orgasmic contractions. The Pulse III also comes in a Duo version for couples with a vibrating underside, and both can be worn flaccid or erect.

Butt plugs are specifically designed to make anal penetration safe and pleasurable, as they have a flared base to ensure that they do not get lost in your beautiful butt. They come in many shapes and sizes and some curve to apply pressure (and vibrations) to the prostate. You will find butt plugs made of silicone, metal, glass, wood, and rubber, and some have external bonuses like sparkly crystals and even furry tails. If you are into butt stuff, you might also want to try out some **anal beads**, which are strung together by a piece of soft rubber with a loop that hangs on the outside. Popping them out can be just as enticing as sliding them in.

If there is one prop that we'd like to see in every bedroom across the nation (and beyond), it is the trusty **blindfold**. Not only can removing your sense of sight heighten your other senses, but it can increase feelings of vulnerability and help you to feel more in the moment as you drown out distractions.

If you are into sensory deprivation, you might also consider exploring sound deprivation and limitation using **gags**. Homemade gags might simply involve a pair of underwear, socks, or stockings you slide into your lover's mouth to minimize sound. Whether you opt for a freshly laundered or a recently worn item, be sure to leave some cloth hanging out for quick removal.

You might also opt for a **cleave gag**, which ties around your head and fits between your teeth, a **bandit-style gag** that covers your mouth and/or nose, or a **ring gag** that fits inside your mouth to keep it open. You can also purchase **ball gags** that are attached to two straps and are either tapered at the back for comfort or perforated to ensure you can breathe.

Whenever you limit your lover's ability to speak, be sure to designate a safe signal and check in regularly to make sure they are comfortable and enjoying the experience. Never leave them unattended when they're gagged, as they need to be within eyesight in order for you to recognize their visual or physical safe signal.

Pain and pleasure go hand in hand, and **clamps** offer the opportunity to explore the hazy pleasure/pain divide. You can purchase clamps designed for specific body parts, but you can also experiment with bobby pins and smooth-edged paper clips on your nipples, labia, areolae, scrotum, thighs, or penis, proceeding very gradually to test your pain thresholds. Other options include nipple suckers, vibrating clamps, or clamps with bells attached to warn your lover of every movement.

Whips and **floggers** have become more common, but some are easier to learn to use than others. Learning to throw a single-tail whip, for example, requires instructions and practice, so consider taking a course online or at your local sex-positive shop or dungeon. Floggers, on the other hand, are usually softer and may be easier to play with for beginners. Composed of multiple flat tails of leather or other materials attached to a short handle, they are usually shorter and softer than whips. Practice with your flogger on a pillow first and then try it very gently on your thigh before proceeding to play with a partner.

Pervertables: Kinky Seduction

The BDSM and kink communities often emphasize the use of various toys and props for sexual stimulation. Everything from handcuffs to electricity tools are used to heighten the sexual tension, kindle desire, and amplify pleasure. Of course, you may not have a dungeon full of props or a chest of toys at your disposal. Whether you identify as a kinkster or not, you can find everyday items in your home to ramp up your sexual pleasure, so consider going on a treasure hunt to see what regular household items can be perverted into sexual accoutrements.

Kinky Items in Your Kitchen:

▶ Wooden spoons, spatulas, and other flat, wide utensils can be used to spank or hit for impact play.

▶ Knives can create a seductive and vulnerable experience when the edges are traced lightly along your skin. Of course, you need to understand the amount of risk you are taking upon yourself when you are engaging in knife play. Ensuring safe words and the ability to opt out of the situation at any given time is a must. We recommend you stay away from major arteries and veins, and if you don't know where they are, we suggest that you avoid knives altogether. ‡

---

‡   It is your responsibility to educate yourself about the risks associated with any form of kink play—including knives, restraints, and other equipment—and to take safety precautions that will allow you to play as safely as possible. For beginners looking to learn more about kink and BDSM, *The Ultimate Guide to Kink: BDSM, Role Play and the Erotic Edge* by Tristan Taormino and *The Ultimate Guide to Bondage: Creating Intimacy Through the Art of Restraint* by Mistress Couple are two great places to start!

▸ Kitchen towels and dish cloths can be stuffed in the mouth as gags to minimize talking as a form of deprivation.

▸ Ice may be utilized for temperature play; trace an ice cube along the body or over the genitals.

▸ Carrots, cucumbers, and other phallic items may be used for oral and vaginal penetration. Be sure to only use them with condoms and lubricant, and do not use them for anal penetration.

▸ Chip clips double as nipple pinchers or skin clamps.

▸ Aprons can be worn to cook nearly naked or used as restraints for a hot bondage scene or role-play.

▸ A variety of kitchen utensils (e.g., forks, spoons, pans) can be used for anticipatory sound play; blindfold your lover and experiment with different sounds to pique their interest and confuse/overwhelm their senses.

▸ Food can be used for olfactory torture and pleasure (e.g., with a blindfold).

▸ Plastic wrap can also be a great way to bind someone, restrict their movement, and admire how their skin looks underneath. Just be sure not to stretch it as you tie up your partner, as you don't want to cut off any circulation.

Kinky Items in Your Bedroom:

▸ Ties and scarves make the perfect restraint tools or blindfolds.

▸ Belts can be used as both restraints and spanking instruments.

▸ Socks can be stuffed in the mouth as gags, and you can kink it up if you like dirty socks.

▸ Clothing can be used to play with gender and cross-dress.

▸ Halloween costumes of all sorts are often used for role-play.

▸ Pillows can be used for sensory deprivation, sound restriction, and a variety of positions.

▸ Bedsheets can be used as restraints.

Kinky Items in Your Bathroom:

▸ Bathtubs, showers, and toilets can be used for golden showers and water sports (pee play).

▸ Mouthwash containing menthol or peppermint oil can be incorporated into oral sex sensation play.

▸ Shaving razors can be used to shave body hair off your partner as part of a kinky or sensual scene.

▸ Combs, brushes, nail files, electric toothbrushes, electric clippers, exfoliating gloves, loofahs, and regular toothbrushes can be used all over the body for sensation play.

▸ Towels and soft sponge poufs double as gags.

▸ Makeup brushes can be used for sensory play and hot wax application.

We encourage you to look around your house for other items that function as pervertables. We are certain that you can find things in the living room or in the garage that help to spark the kinky artist in you. The world is a kinky paradise in hiding, so it's up to you to be creative and uncover the tools needed for a good time!

SEDUCTION INSTRUCTION

Scout out a room in your house that has one or more pervertables. Set up a secret sex date for your lover(s) and lure them into that room. During the seduction phase, grab one of the items out of its proper place and use it on your lover(s) (with consent, of course).

Whether you source seduction and foreplay props in your house or at a specialty store, they are sure to inject creativity and curiosity into your sexual routine. You do not have to buy the whole lot or turn every household item into a pervertable, but if you continue to be open and experimental with tangible objects, you will likely find that they help to keep your sex life fiery for years and decades to come.

SEDUCTION FOR BUSY PEOPLE

If you find that you are too tired, too busy, or too distracted to seduce your lover or be seduced, fret not, as small changes can have a significant impact on your sex life. Sex does not have to be a long, drawn-out experience each and every time, and you don't have to have a specific type of sex in order to reap the benefits of sexual connection. In this chapter, we share specific strategies you can utilize to have more frequent and satisfying sex even when your calendars are full.

If you skipped the chapter on Eroticizing Daily Interactions, we strongly suggest that you go back to it now, as your day-to-day dealings have a greater impact on sexual desire and fulfillment than any technique related to seduction or pleasure. If you previously committed to making changes to your daily interactions, consider whether or not you have been prioritizing and following through or if there are adjustments you can make right now to make your dealings more playful and erotic and to lay the foundation for a hotter sex life.

Important reminder: before you peruse these suggestions for prioritizing sex in the context of a hectic lifestyle, commit to proceeding with an open mind. If you find yourself making excuses for why you can't implement a strategy or why an approach will not work for you, consider whether or not you are really committed to making time for sex and intimacy. It's not uncommon for folks whose lives are privileged in various ways to make excuses by noting that our lives are somehow more difficult than others'. *This won't work because I have three kids and she only has two. If I do this, my wife will just laugh. I can't do this because I work longer hours than him. My partner will never be into this. My job is harder. My family is more demanding. My life is harder.*

We all face personal and relational challenges, but if you have come this far, you know that small changes are manageable and impactful. And the bottom line is that you can make changes or you can make excuses. You cannot do both.

Strategies for Busy Couples

Secretly Schedule Sex

You've probably heard that scheduling sex is essential for busy couples, but many people complain that setting a date and time detracts from the thrill of spontaneity. However, spontaneity is not the norm for most busy people. For the most part, you don't spontaneously eat, drink, or go to a party, so you can't expect sex to be entirely spontaneous either. However, you can balance planning with surprise and cultivate spontaneity by taking turns *secretly* scheduling sex. This means that rather than designating Saturday night as date night, each person plans to initiate sex once per week (or any predetermined period of time). They decide in advance as to when they are going to initiate and make a mental or calendar note to follow through.

This can help to ensure that sex is not entirely predictable and can encourage you to share in the task of initiating sex so that the onus does not fall on one party alone. And though it's not entirely spontaneous, by taking turns with your lover, you each get a "surprise" sex session at some point during the week. You will need to make sure that your schedules align (e.g. do not schedule sex on a Tuesday morning when you know your partner will be working) and be flexible, because plans sometimes change. You might set your alarm half an hour early on Monday to sneak in some morning sex before work, or you might plan an elaborate evening that begins with a sensual massage. The more varied your approaches, the more exciting the experience will be.

SEDUCTION INSTRUCTION

Plan to initiate sex with your partner(s) some time in the next three days. Think about how you will set the scene, approach them, and ensure that you follow through. Set a note in your calendar, ask them to clear their schedule for a date, and do not allow yourself to make excuses. If you are willing to follow through, say it out loud right now: *I've got this. I'll seduce them on Friday.*

Consider Having Sex When You're Not in the Mood

If you wait until you are in the mood for sex, you may never have it. This is because sexual desire does not always arise spontaneously. For some of us, the desire for sex occurs regularly and unprompted by sexual stimuli, but for others, desire is responsive and we need *arousal first* in order to experience desire. Most of us, however, make the mistake of assuming that sexual desire will arise on its own if we're happy, relaxed, and intimately attracted to our partners, which is not always the case.

If you go to work all day, make dinner, clean up, put the kids to bed, listen to your friend complain about their job on the phone, and then hop into bed, you may not experience an intense desire to have sex; you may be more likely to hop into bed pining for sleep. If, however, you go to work all day, make dinner, clean up, put the kids to bed, listen to your friend complain about their job, *and* do something (e.g., fantasize, read an erotic book, touch yourself, ask for a massage) to get aroused, sexual desire may follow.

We're not suggesting that you should have sex if you don't want to, but simply that if you want to want sex, you may need to get aroused in order to open yourself up to the *possibility* of sex—even if you are not in the mood at first.

If you are busy with work, family, and social commitments, you likely need to find shortcuts to arousal in order to experience sexual desire. And if you want to seduce your partner in the context of a busy lifestyle, you will want to get to know their shortcuts to sexual arousal and desire.

Some of these shortcuts for busy people might include:

Consume erotic material. Read your partner a sexy story or underline a few lines from a sexy novel that you would like to share. You can even go to an erotic book reading or attend an erotic show showcasing burlesque and/or erotic poetry.

Fantasize. When was the last time you thought about your partner in a sexual way or daydreamed about your last fun sexual experience? Take the time in the middle of the day (e.g., on your lunch break) and play back a sexual memory from your head. After you have thought about it, text your lover(s) and compliment them or ask them to recall additional details from your shared memory.

Use toys to start your engine. Your partner may not be in the mood initially, but if they're game, a vibrator or stroker may help lead them to arousal and sexual desire. Research reveals that vibrator use is positively correlated with desire, lubrication, orgasm, lower levels of pain, and overall sexual satisfaction.[28]

Give orders and ask your partner to please you. One of the hottest ways to seduce your lover involves being direct. Your partner is not a sexual mind reader, and busy people appreciate when you are straightforward.

For example:

> *I'm exhausted, but I want you. Will you go down on me?*
> *I know we only have a few minutes, but will you finger me to get*
> *me off before I leave for work?*
> *We only have a few minutes alone. Let's . . .*

Take Turns

If you have a partner, don't wait until your sexual moods align to have sex. If you are in the mood and your partner isn't, ask for what you want. Perhaps they will be willing to use their hands, tongue, lips, toys, or other methods to pleasure you. And when the roles are reversed, reciprocate. Heteronormative expectations of sex can lead to both narrow definitions of sex and also problematic expectations with regard to intercourse as the only type of sex that counts. But it doesn't have to be this way. Oral sex, manual sex, sex with a vibrator, rubbing off, watching porn, and a variety of other types of sex can be just as satisfying and do not require that you're both in the mood for one specific activity or outcome.

Try Quickie Seduction Techniques

Sometimes you have time to build seduction over the course

of several hours or days, and other times, you only have a few minutes to squeeze sex in.

Remember that just because you're in the mood for a quickie, that doesn't mean that your partner will be similarly inclined. This is why talking about how you like to be seduced and clarifying your sexual desires is of paramount importance. If you know that your partner isn't into quickies, respect their boundaries. Don't pressure them or suggest that there are universal benefits to quickies on which they are missing out—no sexual activity is a universal fit for every person. You can present and propose any scenario to your partner, but if you pressure them to oblige your needs, you will damage both your sex life and your relationship.

If your partner has communicated that they're not into quickies but you find that time is a scarce commodity, you don't have to give up on quick seduction altogether. Instead, think about how seduction functions over the course of your day or week. Then, talk with your partner(s) about ways that work for them to quickly build arousal, so that you can still connect intimately when time is short.

If you're in a rush and looking for simple ways to initiate sex, consider the following approaches:

▸ Slip into the washroom while they are in the shower. Touch yourself and let them know that peeping on them gets you all riled up. Ask them if you can join them or if you should wait in bed for them. Be very clear about your desire for *your lover* specifically, as opposed to your desire for sex more generally (unless they've already expressed a specific wish to *not* be the object of your desire). Get yourself ready for sex—fantasize, touch yourself, use a vibrator, read a story, watch a video, or give yourself an orgasm first so that your body and mind are in the moment and ready to go when you finally get together. Ask them to do the same.

▸ Hang lingerie, a harness, leather or latex garments, or other undergarments on the back of the bathroom door while they're in the shower or tub. Include a note asking them to join you in the bedroom in their new garb.

▸ Send them a text message from the bedroom (assuming they're in the yard or home office, for instance) and let them know that you're waiting. *I'm waiting and willing to please. I'm naked and ready to go—at your service.* If you are going to interrupt them or take them away from a responsibility, you will likely have more luck if you're clear about your willingness to be generous and take care of their needs first.

▸ Forget rose petals and lingerie. Leave a trail of your favorite lube and toys leading them to the bedroom (or kitchen table, if you are so inclined).

▸ Be demanding. Oftentimes, we assume that our seduction and sexual initiation routine should focus on our partner's pleasure, but prioritizing your own pleasure can be just as appealing—for both of you. Leave them a note on the kitchen counter: *Had a rough day. Don't want to talk. Just want you to touch me/massage me/go down on me/ let me go down on you. You up for it?* Of course, you don't want to pressure your partner. You want to make suggestions and requests and ensure that they feel comfortable doing the same.

Just because you have a small amount of time doesn't mean that you can't be just as erotic as you intend to be. Be thoughtful, be direct, and be a good sport when it comes to being quick!

Sext Seductively

Beguile your lover with suggestive sexts throughout the day or week. Over half of couples use sexting as a prelude to in-person encounters, and the number is on the rise.

Consider your lover's seduction learning style and their core erotic feeling as you craft messages that make them feel sexy, desired, curious, excited, relaxed, challenged, loved, nervous, catered to, enticed, and more. Take advantage of the variety of options available to you, including photos, videos, voice notes, texts, GIFs, and live chats.

Sexting is often depicted as a high-risk activity, but it is low risk in terms of physical outcomes, and you can take precautions to minimize risk of your photos being leaked.

Before you get started, ensure that your partner consents to sexting. Do not be a textual harasser. Consent is mandatory in sex and sexting, so be sure to ask for permission and be mindful of your lover's boundaries. You also want to consider your own risk tolerance, as every photo you take and text might be seen by eyes for which it wasn't intended. And never share a photo of someone else without their clear consent; legal consequences exist for this type of violation.

Once you've ensured consent and considered safety and risk, you're ready to get started . . .

You might **begin with creative language**, including dirty talk phrases expressing what you want to do to please them and to be pleased. This may appeal to those who are auditory and visual, so consider crafting your messages with broad and vivid vocabulary.

If you're meeting someone for the first time or are in a new relationship in which you have mutually consented to exchanging sexy photos, you might limit your personal exposure by **sharing images of your body from the neck down**. By leaving your

face out, you can tempt and titillate a new partner while mini-
mizing your risk of exposure should the photos be leaked. Some
take the extra precaution of adding fake tattoos to their pics, so
that their body is even less recognizable.

If you have a long-term lover whom you trust and you want
to include your face, **use a selfie stick** to get your best angles.
When you're in the mood to snap pics, take a few extra so that
you can send them in the future, and consider using an app that
is separate from their main texting function so that your photos
don't get mixed in with your daily banter.

Part of what makes sexting so intoxicating is the escalation of
eroticism and anticipation. Oftentimes, we make the mistake of
sending too much too soon. You do not need to begin with pics
of your genitals, and it's worth noting that some (many) people
are not specifically turned on by genital close-ups—remember
the less is more approach to seduction. Instead of sending penis
or labia pics, pick another sexy body part and **shoot it from
multiple angles and zoom distances** to encourage them to
create their own visual of what it looks like in its entirety. For
instance, if you want to take a picture of your upper torso, take it
from each side, take it from up top, take it from the bottom, and
take it from other angles that you think are flattering. You might
send a deluge of photos all at once or send one picture per day or
hour to draw the tease out over time.

Practical considerations should be accounted for when taking
sexy photos as well. For example, as we suggested in the section
on Visual Seduction, **tidy up that room.** Clutter can be a huge
distraction even in the background, so make your bed and adjust
your lights so that your partner can home in on your sex appeal
without visual interference.

Generally speaking, **emojis are not sexy**. They can be fun
and playful, and some preliminary research suggests that couples
who text with emojis have more sex, but they do not tend to

complement sexy pics. No one looks at an emoji and goes, "That's a sexy emoji. I really want to be with them now because that emoji is telling me all I need to know about them." Unless you know your lover is turned on by cartoons, save your emojis for your daily communications and allow your words and photos to do the talking when you sext.

Sexting, of course, is not just about images. **Voice notes** allow you to tap into your lover's audial desires. For those of us who are auditory learners, the sound of a lover's voice (even if they are not talking dirty) can be overwhelmingly hot. Use a low, soft voice to tell them what you want to do. Ask them for what you want. Tell them what you've been thinking about. Let them know you want to please them. Convey your desire and desperation for their touch. Build anticipation by sending one sentence at a time over the course of a day or week, and use some of the aforementioned dirty talk lines to guide you.

Video, of course, offers a more interactive means of sexting. You can prerecord short clips of yourself in the dark or engage in live chats. If you are technically inclined, you might string photos together and zoom in over your body parts, and even consider looping audio in over your video file. If you want to keep it simple, record your naked body in movement, film yourself fondling your hot spots, or film an unclear masturbation scene in the dark, allowing your sounds to convey your pleasure. Clips can be as short as a few seconds, so do not feel pressure to produce a professional-quality performance. There's a reason why amateur porn is often more appealing than high-budget films.

And don't forget that you do not have to send videos of yourself; sexy videos and GIFs you come across online can be equally appealing when complemented by a personal note like *We should try this tonight* or *This made me think of you*. You may also opt to film yourself talking to your lover: you might compliment them, tell them how much you enjoyed a recent encounter, tease them by removing clothing (even if they can only see you from the shoulders up) or simply express your love if their core erotic feeling is related to being cared for. You don't have to be sexually explicit to be sexually enticing, so find an approach that suits your style to increase the likelihood of following through.

With photos and voice notes, you may also opt to inundate your partner with multiple messages as you get closer to actually connecting in person. For example, you might send a series of communiqués all at once, or send a variety on multiple platforms—via email, via text, on an app like InTheMood, *and* via private message on social media platforms. This can be particularly appealing to kinesthetic learners who enjoy movement and physical distraction—the next best thing to real-life touch.

If you are sexting with a long-term partner, get creative with your approaches. Send sexy messages while the kids or roommates are in the room. Hit send before you walk in the door at the end of the day. Interrupt their day with an unexpected sext, or change their screensaver to a sexy photo when they leave their phone unattended. Obviously, you will want to be mindful of how they use their phone (e.g., do their coworkers or kids sometimes pick it up to check the time, or do they safeguard it in their bag at all times?) to ensure your safety and privacy and show respect to other folks in your lives.

Digital technology is often painted with broad strokes, and there's no denying that it can detract from intimate connection. However, technology is not the problem—human use (and abuse) ultimately determines its effects. You can use technology to your advantage to make it a healthy component of your relationships, and be sure to set limits on its use to minimize the potential detriments. However you sext, be sure to continuously check in with your partner(s) to ensure that you are respecting their boundaries, as these can change over time depending on living, working, and personal circumstances.

Webcam/Videophone Seduction

Whether you are in a long-distance relationship or experimenting with digi-sex with your live-in partner(s), webcam experiences are among the most vivid and interactive. Live video interactions can be used to build desire, cultivate trust, inject an element of risk, and play various roles that may not be accessible in person.

As with every sexual activity, assess safety and risk factors in the context of your lifestyle and relationship before proceeding with a live video chat, as there is always a possibility of being recorded.

If you are nervous or don't know where to begin with a video chat, you can learn a great deal from signing on to other professional video chat sites. Adult camming is a growing industry that includes some fascinating and novel approaches to interactive sex. You can learn and interact with models of all genders, sexual orientations, skill sets, and proclivities. If you browse a few sites right now, you will see models talking about their weekend, painting their toenails, dancing, playing games, stripping, touching themselves, engaging in partnered sex, and being highly creative with their approaches to both viewer interaction and monetization. Many are adept at ensuring that the buildup escalates over time and allowing their authentic selves to generate intense desire and arousal among their viewers.

You might choose to learn through observation and be inspired by their performances, or you can chime in via the live chat. However you choose to indulge, we strongly encourage you to compensate them for their time if you can afford to do so. Their skills, experience, and knowledge merit respect and recompense.

If you are in a relationship in which signing on to an adult webcam site might violate the terms of your commitment, or if you are unsure how your partner might feel about this, discuss this in advance. You might even consider watching webcam models perform together, and if you do, consider how this fits into the boundaries and expectations of your relationship. Some questions to generate reflection and discussion include:

▶ If we do this together, does it mean we can do it alone? Set parameters and agree upon what is acceptable within the confines of your relationship. Don't worry about what others (including experts) have to say. You decide what is dis/allowed in your own relationship as a team.

▶ Are we willing to interact (chat) with the models, or just watch?

▶ Are you nervous about the experience? What makes you nervous? What can your partner do to assuage your concerns?

▶ If you feel uncomfortable at any point, how will you address this? Will you close the computer? Take a break? Will you use a sign to communicate your discomfort?

▶ If you're using a pay site (many offer free access), what spending limit do you want to set?

Be honest about your desires and boundaries. You are not a prude if you're not into adult webcams, and you don't have to do *everything* to have a happy relationship and satisfying sex life.

Should you choose to proceed with webcam seduction on your own, begin by clearing the background, adjusting the lights, wiping down your camera (unless you want it to be blurry), selecting a flattering angle, and assuming a comfortable position that can be maintained over a period of time. Cam models will tell you that rookies often make the mistake of setting the camera at an angle that flatters their initial positioning, but don't realize how tiring the position can be. Prioritize your comfort.

Because you will be able to see your camera's view on your screen (if you're using a computer), take a moment to minimize (or hide) this portion of your view so that you do not stare at yourself throughout the experience and can make eye contact with your camera.

You can begin by simply talking. Ask them what they want to do. What do they want to see? What do they want to hear? Listen, give positive feedback, and validate their desires with smiles, giggles, nods, *ahh*s, *mm-hmm*s, and deep breaths. Ask specific questions to drill into the finer details of their desires.

Share your desires too. What are you thinking about? How are you feeling? What do you feel in your body? What do you want to see? What do you want to hear? Do you have any special requests? Remember that seduction is not only about your performance, but also includes actively pursuing your own desires.

When you're feeling turned on, you may slowly start to undress. It can be effective to wear multiple layers to build anticipation and keep them curious. Be sure to cultivate consent as you proceed.

As you undress, ask them how they're feeling. Inquire as to what they're feeling. Ask them to show you a specific body part or movement. Let them know what is coming next and what you want from them in order to make it happen. For example, *if you show me yours, I'll show you mine*, or *I want to touch myself, but I want to see you undress first.*

You can play the role of director or pupil—whichever suits you best. If you want to direct your partner, give specific instructions: *Touch your nipple with your thumb. Lick your thumb and rub it all around. Slower. Now look up at me. Lick your lips. Turn your head to the side so I can see your tongue along your lips. Suck your finger into your mouth. Now come a little closer. I want to see you up close. Can you blow me a kiss? Taste yourself for me. Reach down and let me watch you get your fingers wet. Now rub them along your cheek. Keep rubbing. Now suck them in. How do you taste? Tell me how you taste. Do you want me to taste you?*

You might also talk about what you might do if you were in the room with them (as a fantasy). *I'm going to come over. Do you want me to? Would you wait for me? Can I touch you? Can I slide my fingers inside you? How much can you take? I want to help you get a taste, but first I want to touch your entire body. I want to smell you and taste you from head to toe. I'm coming over to suck you off.*

Or you can talk about how you are feeling. *I want it so badly. I wish you were here to take care of me. I can feel the juices on my legs. Can you see them? My nipples hurt, I want you to suck them so badly. I'm aching for you. I'm going to touch myself. It feels so good. My fingers are cold, and this makes my body tingle. It's too much.*

As evidenced by the diversity of profitable content on professional adult webcam sites, there is no right way to use webcams for sexual seduction. You might use them while you're in the next room, or you might use them while you and your partner are in different countries. You can use a webcam for sixty seconds at noon to give your lover a taste of what's to come when you both get home, or you can draw out the experience over the course of a full hour. Some folks use webcams almost every day, and others save them for special occasions. You might prefer to center the shot so that your partner can see everything, or you might opt to position yourself almost entirely off-screen so that your lover has to fill in the visual blanks on their own. You can use the webcam to connect with your one true love or to orchestrate a group orgy with no risk of fluid transmission and no pressure to spend the night.

SEDUCTION INSTRUCTION

If you have yet to utilize video to seduce a lover, there is no better time than the present. Turn on your webcam now and enjoy an offline solo session to get accustomed to being on camera. Turn your Wi-Fi and data off and take a few minutes to play with your body, talk dirty, breathe with desire, and experiment on your own.

Mindful Touch and Seduction for Busy People: How to Manage Distractions

If your lifestyle is fast-paced and hectic, your mind likely wanders during seduction and foreplay (and all sexual activities), and you are not alone. Seduction and sexual pleasure are often hindered by distractions, intrusive thoughts, and/or the pressure of performance. And it is no surprise that we struggle to be present during sex given that sleep deprivation, overcommitment, and the consumption of thirty-four gigabytes of daily data have become the individual norm. You may have unknowingly trained yourself to be distracted by scrolling through filtered images, multitasking (AKA dividing your focus) to save time, and bringing your newsfeed into your bedroom.

But it doesn't have to be this way. You can unlearn these distracting habits and train yourself to be more present in your sexual interactions and relationships through the practice of mindfulness—in and out of the bedroom.

Through the practice of mindfulness, you can overhaul your

default setting so that it no longer involves dividing your attention or using distractions to achieve a specific objective. Instead, you will find that being in the moment and embracing your current emotions and sensations becomes the norm.

Being mindful refers to being engaged in the present experience free from judgment and pressure. It involves showing up for yourself and your partner(s). And when it comes to sex, being mindful precipitates multiple benefits, including heightened desire, greater confidence, lower performance anxiety, and improved sexual functioning including arousal, erection, ejaculatory control, and orgasm. When you are present and mindful, you become more alert and energized, more creative, more connected with yourself, and more connected to your partner.

If you would like to be more in the moment and cultivate a more mindful sexual experience, consider these approaches and activities to get started:

Change the Way You Breathe

When you feel overwhelmed or unable to stay in the moment, calm your body and mind by bringing your focus to your breath. Pay attention to the way the air feels as you inhale through your nose, and take note of the sensations as you exhale slowly through your mouth.

Inhale for 1-2-3-4-5.
Hold for 1-2-3.
Exhale for 1-2-3-4-5.

Repeat five times, and notice how your breath affects your heart rate and emotional state. You are unlikely to use this approach in the middle of a sexual encounter, but it can help to prime your body for sexual desire. You can also use it if you find you need a break during sexual activity.

Aside from cultivating presence, your breath plays a role in your sexual response and pleasure.

During sex, you likely hold your breath for a variety of reasons: nerves, excitement, fear of losing control, an attempt to dampen your sounds so as not to disturb the kids, roommates, or neighbors. You may hold your breath because the heavy breathing that precedes and accompanies orgasm feels unnatural—though it is quite the opposite, as this deep breathing can intensify orgasm. Interestingly, we do the same when we're lifting weights. We hold our breath because we think it gives us more control or strength when, in fact, it limits the oxygen to our system, which can cause our muscles to tire more easily. In both sex and exercise, stifling our breath is counterproductive. When you breathe purposefully and mindfully, you're more likely to feel connected to your body and relish in its pleasurable sensations.

Breathe in a Cloud

Your breath is not only essential to sexual response, but breathing purposefully can help you to be more mindful and connected to your body. The cloud breathing technique combines both breath work and visualization to create a more meaningful connection between your mind and body.

The technique is simple: envision yourself surrounded by a soft, warm, cozy, fluffy cloud. As you inhale, visualize the cloud shrinking around your body. As you exhale, visualize the cloud expanding. As you visualize the cloud enveloping your body, take comfort in imagining its warmth and soft touch.

Continue to inhale while visualizing the cloud closing in on your body and exhale as it expands ever so slightly. You might take six deep breaths when you get into bed or use this approach to be more present throughout the day.

As you relax into this visualization and breathing technique, pay attention to how your body feels in terms of tension and relaxation, temperature, heart rate, weight, texture against your clothing or bedsheets, and general comfort to practice being more mindful of your body's unique responses.

Cloud breathing is not intended to be erotic, and most people do not use it *during* sexual activity, but its practice fosters presence and mindfulness to create a connection between your breath and body. Learning to be mindful of your body and breath *outside* the bedroom will help you to be more mindful in a similar fashion during sexual experiences. You may also find this activity helpful when you first get into bed, if you find you are distracted or distressed by intrusive thoughts; as you focus on your body and breath via the cloud visualization, you will be more present with yourself and better prepared to connect with your body and your partner—however you choose to seduce one another.

Try Mindful Masturbation

Oftentimes we treat self-pleasure sessions as mindless tune-ups and rush through without truly appreciating the full erotic capacity of our bodies. Since most of us learn about our body's sexual response through masturbation, hastening the experience can create bad habits and establish an association between sex and expediency. The practice of mindful masturbation can help you to break these habits, prolong the adventure, and be more conscious of erotic pleasure.

To be more mindful when you masturbate, consider taking orgasm out of the equation. Touch yourself for pleasure for fifteen to twenty minutes *without* trying to reach orgasm. Explore your entire body with your hands, using lube, massage oil, toys, and/or objects of various textures. As you get in touch with your body's distinct responses and breathing patterns, you will find that your ability to stay present during sex (partnered and solo) increases, as you will be less hung up on the performance and more focused on the pleasure itself.

You may also want to experiment with different breathing patterns while you masturbate.

Pay attention to the way you breathe before orgasm and try to draw the breaths out a bit longer to see how it changes the sensations. Some people close their eyes and visualize sending the oxygen to their pelvic region (like in yoga or Pilates), and they say that this sometimes precipitates a state of euphoria—an oxygen high.

Others report that deep, slow breaths extend the orgasmic contractions and make them more intense, so they focus on breathing in through the nose and out through the mouth. Practicing while you masturbate will help normalize the breathing pattern so that eventually it doesn't require focus/effort.

Of course, it's important to note that each person's experience with breathing patterns and pleasure is unique. We've also had clients who find that holding their breath for a short period of time triggers orgasm, so experiment with different breathing patterns to see what works for you.

Engage in a Digital Detox

Each night, lock your phones and tablets away. Put them in the basement, car, or a kitchen cupboard. Designate a specific time and set an alarm in your calendar so that you follow through. If you don't want to do this every night, begin with one night per week and add a second night in a few weeks.

Make an effort to fall asleep and wake up to your lover, as opposed to checking in with your online friends as soon as you open your eyes. If your phone is your alarm clock, invest in an actual alarm clock and stop making excuses.

Once you become accustomed to nightly detoxes, consider adding tech-free time to your weekly or daily routine. Perhaps you opt to leave your phone in the trunk whenever you hop in the car, or you might choose to have phone-free dinners several times per week. Some couples we work with designate one hour after work as tech-free (they leave their phones in their cars or bags) so that they have time to reconnect and catch up after a busy day. And other families put their phones and tablets in a box in the closet before dinner—this can be helpful whether you are dining solo, with a partner, or in a group.

Whatever limits you set for your digital detox, consider keeping track of how you feel while you're tech-free. Compare your degree of presence on the days in which you abstain from technology to those in which you indulge without limits.

Chart for tracking:

Did I take a digital detox today? Yes/No
Note on what this digital detox entailed:
I feel good about my body. Scale of 1-10
I feel connected to my body. Scale of 1-10
I feel physically at ease. Scale of 1-10
I feel emotionally at ease. Scale of 1-10
I feel close to my partner/other loved ones. Scale of 1-10
I feel in the moment and present. Scale of 1-10

Focus on One Sense to Engage in Sensual Presence

When you tap into your senses, it brings you back to the present moment. You cannot *smell* in the future or *hear* in the past. You can only see, taste, hear, smell, and touch in the present.

To practice sensual presence, home in on one sense, like your sense of sound. Close your eyes. Tune into the most obvious sounds you hear right now. Take a few slow breaths and then deepen your listening. What else do you hear in the distance? Breathe as you embrace these sounds. Notice their finer details—their volume, rhythm, and vibrations. What do you feel in your body as you listen?

As you learn to be mindful in your everyday life, being present and open to sensual pleasure will become more natural, as will being mindful about the way you interact with and seduce your lover(s). Try a few minutes of sensual presence before you walk in the door at night, and see how you respond differently to those you love.

Deprive Yourself (or Your Partner)

Lower the lights, close your eyes, wear a blindfold, or invest in sound-canceling headphones to help you to be more mindful and focus on sex when you are busy or distracted. The deprivation of one sense can heighten another, which can help you to focus on your lover's touch, voice, appearance, or scent—and this can lead to a more mindful connection and heightened attraction.

This approach can be particularly useful if you are trying to seduce a partner who finds themselves easily distracted. They may want to experience sexual pleasure, but struggle to stay in the moment, and they may ask for your help getting in the mood. Of course, it's not your job to put them in the mood all the time (they have to make the lifestyle, attitudinal, and behavioral adjustments if they want to want sex), but you can lend a hand via sensory deprivation.

Ask them if they are open to being blindfolded while you touch their body.

Ask them if they'd like to wear earplugs, plug in a white-noise machine, or play loud music to drown out distracting sounds while you touch their body for pleasure.

Offer them the option of lying in the dark while you whisper in their ear or read them a story that turns them on.

Sometimes managing distractions is not only about focusing on the present, but eliminating one sensory stimulus so that you can tune into another.

Put Intrusive Thoughts in a Box

If you find that thoughts of work, kids, or upcoming responsibilities detract from your ability to get in the mood, try a visualization exercise in which you place these troublesome thoughts in a box. Picture yourself shelving the box away outside your room (e.g., in the garage or closet), so that you can return to it at a later time.

If the thought returns, don't stress. Accept it and remind yourself that the worry, concern, or issue is waiting for you in a box and you can address it tomorrow. Take a few breaths to recenter yourself and bring your attention to your partner's touch, or listen to the sound of their breath.

It's normal to experience intrusive thoughts even when you are thoroughly enjoying a sexual experience. As we mentioned earlier with reference to the white bears, there's no point in attempting to banish a thought (it has the opposite of the intended effect); acknowledge it without judgment, put it away, and tune into one of your senses to bring yourself back to the present moment.

Try the Face Caress with a Partner

You may not consider your face an erogenous zone, but the skin on your cheeks, chin, and forehead tends to be highly responsive to sensual touch. The face caress involves touching, feeling, and kissing your lover's face for five to ten minutes. Take turns being the giver and receiver, and be sure to use your fingertips, palms, lips, breath, and the backs of your hands as you explore every contour of their face.

When it's your turn to receive touch, breathe deeply and allow yourself to enjoy the relaxation and indulgence of a sensual face massage intended to please and pamper.

Touch for pleasure and connection with no specific goal or outcome. Be mindful of the texture, temperature, stroke, pressure, and rhythm of your lover's touch.

When you are done, take a few minutes to hold hands, spoon, and/or breathe in sync.

SEDUCTION INSTRUCTION

These mindfulness practices not only improve sex, but also deepen the connection we experience with the one(s) we love. Being mindful can help us to tune into our own emotions and recognize our lover's feelings, vulnerabilities, and needs. Consider how you can be more mindful right now. Can you close your eyes and tune into one physical sensation in your body? Perhaps you feel your body against the cushion or mattress or your feet against the floor. If you're reading this book in a park (good for you!) or under a fan, can you feel the wind or air against your skin? Pay attention to the most obvious sensation and then tune in a little more intently to pick up on the less obvious ones. Take a few breaths as you home in on your sense of touch. How do you feel in your body? Are you comfortable? Can you shift around to improve your comfort? Are any of your muscles tense? Does adjusting your position help them to relax and be at ease? Even two minutes of mindfulness can help you to feel more connected to yourself, your body, and your environment. Developing this practice outside of the bedroom will help the experience arise more naturally when you are aroused.

A note on mindfulness as social lubrication: As you read through these mindfulness exercises and seduction techniques, you might have assumed that getting intoxicated will facilitate or enhance your performance. And while a drink or toke may help you to relax and loosen up, too much of a good thing can lead to miscommunication and regret. (Having said this, you know your body and its response to substances best, so you can determine how much to use and how to reduce harm when you do.). It is worth noting that the practice of mindfulness can be as effective at lowering inhibitions and self-consciousness as any intoxicating substance, without the hangover, apologies, and regret. It can help you to feel more grounded, heighten your connection to your body, and augment self-confidence.

We've only scratched the surface with regard to mindful sex, and we encourage you to keep exploring. You might download a general mindfulness app to begin and end each day mindfully or read up on mindful sex (we suggest Laurie Brotto's *Better Sex Through Mindfulness*, which explores both theories and real-life stories). If you want a guided approach to mindfulness exercises designed to benefit your relationship and sex life, check out the Mindful Sex video course hosted by me (Jess) and Dr. Reece Malone (available at HappierCouples.com).

Online Seduction

Seduction no longer begins when you meet in person, as you can now choose from thousands of apps and programs related to online dating and mating—many of which are free to use. Digital dating has altered the sex and relationship landscape and has changed the ways in which we communicate and interact with potential partners. Some people consider this change primarily positive, as you can now meet more people than ever from all corners of the world. Others lament the loss of community-based connections and consider the so-called old-fashioned way more simple, easy, and straightforward. We believe that there are benefits to all approaches and suggest that you can blend digital and in-person dating and seduction to suit your needs.

If you're interested in exploring online dating or improving your online seduction approach, consider the following strategies. They are all rooted in being more authentic in order to attract partners well suited to your needs and to filter out those interested in playing games.

Present a clear picture of your face(s) and consider smiling. If you like to smile, let it shine. Research and common sense confirms that a genuine smile makes you more attractive, as you appear healthier, more confident, and approachable. Some folks use blurry or filtered images to distort their appearance and/or age, but we suggest that you use a photo that reflects your true appearance. Select a shot in which you appear attractive and don't use a photo that reflects what you looked like two, five, or ten years ago. You want to put your best foot forward *and* attract someone who is drawn to the real you.

If you're single and looking for a date, don't include friends in your profile photo, as daters do not want to play a guessing game or be tasked with scrolling through all of your photos to figure out who you are. Online dating moves quickly, and most daters are not going to take the time to do detective work, so make it easy for them to recognize what you look like from the outset. If you are a couple looking for a date, choose a profile photo that shows both of your faces and reflects your love and affection for one another.

Supplement your profile photo with additional pictures so that folks who are attracted to your main photo can get to know a little about you via visual representation. Post at least five photos to give them the opportunity to learn about the things you value. Do you have kids or pets? Do you like to dance or hike? Do you like cosplay or kink? Share these values and preferences in your photo album. Of course, if you believe your job might be adversely affected by your public profile, err on the side of caution if your (culturally) subversive desires and values might put you at risk.

As you craft your profile, highlight information about the person you are, as opposed to the person you want to be. **What identities do you hold and cherish for yourself?** Mention your identities that are important to you, and let the person decide if those identities are compatible with their desires.

List your hobbies and interests and be honest about how you spend your time. Are you into traveling to foreign countries? Do you love drinking and dancing at the club? Do you spend your spare time hiking and camping new trails? Describe the type of person you are. Is your horoscope sign important to you? Mention it. Is physical fitness a must? Share the types of physical activities you enjoy. Are you a smoker or social drinker? Make it known.

Feel free to **share a few details about what you're looking for** as well. Do you want someone who loves to travel and is open to living and moving around the world at some point? Are you looking for a partner who loves theater and the arts? Share this from the onset so that others can self-select, and remember that a missed connection is not personal—they simply may not be a good fit.

Do not be afraid to **acknowledge your perceived flaws and limitations**. Is there something about you that you think would turn some people off? Feel free to share it. Although this may seem counterintuitive when it comes to seduction and attraction, it can be helpful. Admitting to shortcomings shows vulnerability, which is often a reflection of trust and confidence. Are you a procrastinator? Are you always late? Consider mentioning these traits and habits in your profile, so that people can either decide that you won't be a good fit or benefit from seeing themselves in you.

As you share your strengths, interests, and even a few vulnerabilities, **do not reveal everything about yourself**. Mystery breeds curiosity, so save something for your potential in-person meeting. You begin dating online, but you do not want to end the connection online. If you're messaging with a potential date, **limit the number of messages you exchange** (e.g., we set our limit to seven, others limit themselves to fifteen) or predetermine how long you are willing to chat online before meeting in person. Share these self-imposed guidelines with your chat mates and use them to motivate yourself to take action rather than waiting for them to initiate further contact. (e.g., *I have a rule for myself that if we've been chatting for two weeks, we should try to meet in person. Are you up for it?*)

When you connect with someone online, **be honest about your expectations** and ask them to clearly state their intentions. Do you want a relationship or a casual hookup? Do you get emotionally attached after sex or do you see sex as a carnal act? Do you want monogamy, consensual nonmonogamy, or are you open to multiple arrangements? Be honest with yourself first so that you can convey your desires to your dates.

As you peruse online profiles, try to **engage beyond their initial photo.** Folks complain that online dating (and the swiping culture, in particular) is superficial, but they engage in superficial dating themselves by swiping away too quickly. Can you defy these norms and take a few minutes to read through profiles *before* you make a declaration about (a lack of) chemistry or attraction? Both attraction and chemistry can be cultivated over time, and in long-term relationships, you will be forced to invest in this cultivation, so it's a good habit to establish from the onset.

When you decide to message a potential date (please do not feel you have to wait for others to message you), open with a few lines that indicate that you have read their profile (*I see you're a hiker too. I'm new to it, but I'm really liking it and I'm going to Valley of Fire next month. Have you been there, or do you have any trail tips?*). Be curious and complimentary (e.g., *I love that pic of you at Antelope Canyon*). Ask them about something they wrote, and don't open with generic phrases (e.g., *Hi. How's it going?*). Show genuine interest, and you will be rewarded with the same in return (if they are a good fit for you).

Remember that **rejection is a part of life**. If you try to avoid it, you will always live in fear. The most powerful, successful, attractive, and admirable people in the world have faced rejection and continue to embrace it every single day. You are worthy of love *and* you will face rejection, so accept it, enjoy the challenge, and continue to learn from your experiences.

If you are curious about online dating, but don't know how to get started, **enlist a friend to help you**. They can lend a hand writing your dating profile, select your photos, and set up your account. Those in monogamous relationships might be particularly keen to assist, as they may be drawn to living vicariously through your new and exciting dating experiences.

SEDUCTION INSTRUCTION

Take three to five new pictures that reflect your current lifestyle. Download a dating app that you have never used before and create a thorough profile with the help of a friend. Find a few folks you're interested in messaging and initiate contact. Inject something humorous, cute, or flattering in your message. Show your curiosity. See how many messages you get back, bearing in mind that you do not have to date or commit to anyone today.

16

SEDUCTION AND FOREPLAY GAMES

Sometimes you want to dive right into sex, and other times, you want to be playful and experiment with novel approaches. If you find that your routine is repetitive or predictable, break the cycle by trying out one of these simple games with your lover. Even a few minutes of something new can help to break the autopilot mode so often experienced in long-term relationships and lead to new discoveries.

As always, these activities come with guidelines as opposed to rules, and just like sex, you can always adapt them or make them up as you go.

The Dirty Drip

Combining food and sex is a common fantasy and indulgence, as they both evoke pleasure and activate a similar brain response. Because this activity is a little messy, it's sure to lead to a little laughter and playful affection.

Play by play:

▶ Strip down to a state of undress with which you're comfortable, bearing in mind that you might spill food on whatever garments remain.

▶ Don a blindfold and sit in front of your lover.

▶ Your task is to feed them something delicious (e.g., whipped cream, whipped mascarpone, ice cream, cake icing, honey, chocolate sauce) while blindfolded. If anything spills or drips on them, you agree to lick it up (or use your hands) with their guidance as you remain blindfolded.

Pick a Card

A little forethought goes a long way, so get creative with a range of sex acts to remind yourself of your old favorites or discover new approaches you've yet to try.

Play by play:

▶ Write down as many sexual activities as you can come up with on cue cards (one sex act per card). Nothing is too mild or wild, as you will have a chance to choose activities that appeal to you, and you will always check in to get enthusiastic consent before proceeding. Some varied suggestions from our clients include:

- *Eat ice cream off my breasts*
- *Call me "daddy"*
- *Kiss my neck*
- *Look up at me while you go down on me*
- *Blindfold me and give me a full-body massage*
- *Rub my feet*

- *Put a finger up my butt during oral sex*
- *Kiss me when I'm coming*
- *Suck on my earlobes*
- *Nibble on my lower lip*
- *Let me bite you*
- *Pretend I'm your escort and pay me for sex*
- *Ride me on the kitchen counter*
- *Pull my hair and drag me to bed*
- *Bite my nipples while you caress my face*
- *Cover my mouth with your hand while we're having sex (leave space to breathe through the nostrils)*
- *Try a full-body slide with oil*
- *Massage my butt for twenty minutes with coconut oil*
- *Go down on me while I'm eating a burger at the kitchen table*
- *Gag while you suck on me*
- *Sit on my face with your full body weight*
- *Lick and kiss my bum*
- *Kiss in the dark for five minutes*
- *Spank me (focus on the meaty part of the butt and start slow)*
- *Tie me up (leave space for circulation)*
- *Gag me with your underwear (be sure to leave some space to breathe and leave some fabric hanging out so that it can be removed with ease)*
- *Shove your fingers in my mouth*
- *Lick my [genitals] for ten minutes without talking*

- *Rub my fluids all over your face*
- *Make out with me after you go down on me*
- *Fist me*
- *Suck on my toes*
- *Worship my boots*
- *Paint my toenails*
- *Pee on my back*
- *Put your nose in my butt*
- *Tell me you love me while you go down on me*
- *Eat out my belly button*
- *Have sex on the balcony*
- *Go down on me while I'm on a call with clients*

▶ Once you've built a collection of twenty-plus cards, pick three that you would like to explore further.

▶ Have your partner pick one of your cards, and if you both agree, they have twenty-four hours to bring the sex act to life. They can start right now, if you have time, or you can pull cards right before you leave for work so that you're forced to wait and build anticipation.

▶ Change it up the following week so that you both get to pick a card and initiate a creative sexual activity.

Mirror-Mirror

Explore one another's bodies while depriving yourselves of sight to heighten your other senses and be more mindful of the physical and emotional experience of your lover's touch.

Play by play:

▶ Lie on the bed or sit facing one another. Close your eyes or use scarves as blindfolds.

▶ Take turns touching one another and mirroring one another's actions.

▶ Perhaps you stroke your lover along their collarbone using the backs of your hands; though they cannot see exactly what you are doing, they will try to mimic your movement and touch.

▶ They might suck on their finger and then trace the wet tip between your lips; your job is to repeat the same action.

▶ You may want to experiment with having off-limits areas for a few minutes (e.g., no breast or genital touching), or limit the ways in which you can touch (e.g., can only use the index and middle fingers of your left hand and your breath).

▶ Alternatively, you could place a pile of toys and props between you (e.g., feathers, lube, vibrators, massage oil) and try to mirror your partner using props without the sense of sight.

Party Vibes

Play by play:

▶ The next time you are going to a party, wear a toy that can be hidden beneath your clothing and controlled via remote control or an app on your phone. Some options for the vagina include the We-Vibe Jive or Moxie, which connect to the WeConnect app on your phone or can be controlled via a Bluetooth remote. If you prefer an external panty vibe, **OhMiBod's Club Vibe** is controlled from a remote control. Options for anal play include the **We-Vibe Ditto** and the **Nexus Ace**.

▶ Hand over the reins of control to your lover and discuss your limits, concerns, and desires ahead of time. You might want to pick a signal to use if you want to take a break or call it quits (e.g., you remove your sweater, they should check in with you privately, or if you tap them on the bum, they should turn off the vibrations to allow you to regroup).

▶ Choose a code word or occurrence, and each time your lover encounters it, they agree to turn on, increase, or adjust the intensity of your toy's vibrations. For example, they might do so every time someone says *drink* or each time they shake hands with someone new.

▶ You can play this game to rile one another up (you can both wear separate toys if you have access to them), or you may opt to sneak away to play in person at the party or in your car.

Vibrator use is not only positively correlated with improved sexual functioning, but also with healthy behaviors. One large-scale study conducted by the Kinsey Institute found that women who use vibrators are more likely to have had a gynecological exam, which screens for a number of health issues, including cancer.

Better Than Dice

You've probably come across sexy dice that list body parts and actions on each of their six sides. This game allows you to multiply the sexy dice approach by experimenting with a greater number of body parts and acts as you create your own combinations.

Play by play:

▶ To prepare, gather thirty-plus small pieces of scrap paper, some pens, and two bags or envelopes.

▶ Write down as many body parts as you can come up with, listing one per sheet of scrap paper: lips, nipples, fingers, toes, thighs, neck, lower back, shoulder blades, collarbone, belly button, ankles, backs of knees, hips, clitoris (if one of you has one), penis (if one of you has one), chest, cheeks, forehead, eyelids, calves, etc.

▶ Write down as many erotic verbs/actions as you can think of, listing one per sheet of paper: lick, suck, caress, tickle, nibble, bite, fondle, titillate, vibrate, swirl, stroke, eat, swallow, tease, breathe, blow, taste, rub, etc.

▶ Place the papers listing body parts in one envelope and those listing the actions in the other.

▶ Without peeking, pull out one action paper and one body part paper. Have your lover do the same.

▶ You can opt to perform the action on the body part listed (to yourself or your lover), or you can trade one or both sheets of paper with your lover. Have fun negotiating, touching, and playing with various combinations.

▶ If you prefer to make things more complicated, pull two actions and one body part and experiment with multiple approaches to touch in one area. You may also want to use specific techniques from the Erotic Touch Techniques section instead of more general actions.

Come Closer

If you find that your foreplay game has become routine or that you rush into sex, this activity can help you to slow down and prolong the buildup. Tease your lover and make them quiver with desire by combining elements of trivia and red light, green light.

Play by play:

▶ Sit or lie in bed in whatever state of (un)dress makes you feel sexy and comfortable. Have your lover stand as far away from the bed as possible.

▶ Quiz your lover and allow them to take one step closer each time they get a correct answer. Punish them by having them take a step back when they get an answer wrong. You are the judge, and your ruling stands (even if it's not accurate—this is just for fun).

▶ You can ask them personal questions to see how well they know you or how much they remember about the relationship (e.g., *Where did we first kiss? How old was I when I had my first kiss? What's my favorite ice cream flavor? What color is my go-to sex toy? What brand of lube do I buy? What's my record for number of orgasms? What's my favorite position?*).

▶ Alternatively, you can ask them questions to learn more about what they think and arbitrarily decide if you will accept the answer as correct (e.g., *What do you love most about my body? What's your favorite position? What do you want me to do when you're coming? Where is the hottest place we've had sex? What's the best part of our sex life? What did you fantasize about the last time you masturbated?*) Keep the questions light and playful. There are no right or wrong answers.

▶ Or you might pick real trivia questions from a board game or an app. It's up to you.

> ▶ **While you ask them questions, play with yourself. Use your hands or a vibrator and let them watch. Get yourself turned on, and feel free to have an orgasm if the mood strikes you.** They have to wait until you say they can take another step before proceeding.

> ▶ This game simply allows you to build sexual tension while delaying physical touch, and it can be sexy to feel exposed and even a bit uncomfortable. You might even tap into a new elevated erotic feeling!

Netflix and Strip

Netflix and chill may be the norm when you first meet, but as the months go by, your chill often becomes more literal and less erotic. Rather than binge-watching and falling asleep, get creative with your content consumption and play a strip game while you binge. Agree to remove a piece of your partner's clothing whenever you hear a specific word on-screen. You should each pick a different word and try to select words that will occur with some frequency (i.e., don't pick obscure words like "pig" unless you are watching *Peppa Pig*). For example, if your selected word is yes, you remove one piece of your partner's clothing each time you hear it. If they select no as their magic word, they strip you of one article each time they hear it.

You can share your words, or keep them a secret and let your partner guess. If you don't reveal your word to your lover, it also makes it easier to cheat—and a little cheating is okay in this case, as long as it is playful and consensual.

HOW TO BE SEDUCED

Mastering the art of seduction involves learning to be both a giver and taker. The desire to be a *giver* in bed is admirable, but it is equally important to indulge in receiving pleasure—for your own sake as well as for your lover's. As we've discussed, as you learn to be a *taker*, you will likely feel more physically connected to your body, experience a boost in self-esteem, and provide your partner with the opportunity to embrace the joy and fulfillment of giving.

To improve your capacity to be seduced, be honest about your needs, boundaries, and desires. Some of the exercises in this book (e.g., The Seduction Interview) can help you to evaluate your own needs and convey them to your partner(s), so revisit and update your answers often.

Address your own seduction *accelerants* and *impediments*—the things that make you more open to seduction and those that turn you off. Be clear about these with your lover(s) and take some time to consider why these impediments exist. Your lover(s) can learn to avoid them, but you can also address and eradicate them in some cases.

For example, if hearing your roommates or kids in the next room causes you to shut down any attempts at seduction, can you use a white-noise app to drown out the sounds? If you find that you reject all advances because your mood sours after talking to your brother, can you set boundaries so that you do not take his calls in the evening? Conveying your needs to your lover(s) is essential, but you can also make adjustments to remove some of the seduction impediments in your own life.

Alongside communication and practical lifestyle modifications, you can also learn to be a better taker by **practicing the receipt of physical touch**.

SEDUCTION INSTRUCTION: BE A TAKER

Set aside twenty minutes free from distractions. Ensure that the space is comfortable and private before you adjust the lighting, temperature, and furniture to your liking. You can undress or wear light clothing. Find a comfortable position and start to tune into your breath. Get ready to *receive* pleasure for twenty minutes. Your only job is to breathe and enjoy your lover's touch as they explore your body with their lips, breath, fingertips, and more. Agree in advance that they will spend the full twenty minutes touching your entire body with the exception of the genitals and/or any other hot spot that tends to lead to orgasm. (You can always follow up with orgasm when you're done.)

While engaging in the role of the *taker*, try to focus on how your partner's touch feels in terms of rhythm, pressure, stroke, temperature, and speed. If your mind wanders away from the present moment, notice the distraction without judgment, and try to bring yourself back to the present by focusing on your breath for four inhales and exhales.

You might find that the experience of taking pleasure is particularly challenging—especially if your erotic script is tied to personal performance. But as you learn to be a better taker, you will also become more present and mindful of sex as a powerful experience, as opposed to a performative production.

Carve out time to engage in this twenty-minute activity this week. If Oprah (or one of your idols) called and invited you to lunch, you would find the time, so prioritize yourself above Oprah (unless Oprah calls, in which case you might want to take the call) and make it happen.

The practice of **sexual self-care** can also guide you in the direction of learning to be seduced, but self-care isn't just about bubble baths and spa days. Self-care refers to any practice or mindset that allows you to feel comfortable with yourself and your body. Self-love and self-care are essential to your overall health and well-being. You set the tone for how you expect to be loved by others, so it's important to care for yourself physically, emotionally, psychologically, and (for many people) spiritually.

Sexual self-love is only one component of self-love, but for many of us, it is an important one. How you care for yourself sexually influences how your partner(s) relate(s) to you. Sexual self-love might involve self-pleasure (masturbation) as well as developing a positive body image, effective communication skills, and the ability to release sexual shame.

Some of the benefits of sexual self-love might include:

Improved sexual functioning. Self-pleasure can help you to become more familiar with your own body and its unique sexual responses. You will likely become better at asking for what you want during partnered sex as a result of your self-pleasure sessions.

The relinquishment of sexual shame. Most of us learn to orgasm through self-pleasure, and accepting the fact that orgasm is an *experience* as opposed to something a lover can give you can work wonders for how you see sex and your body.

Boosted body confidence. Masturbation not only fosters a positive connection with your body, but it can boost self-esteem. When your body performs for you, you tend to focus on its strong points as opposed to its "problems."

Heightened sexual desire. Masturbation is elemental to increasing desire in many cases, as it helps us to learn about our own bodies and reactions. Moreover, as your body relishes in the dopamine and endorphin release, you are more likely to crave even more, resulting in an increase in desire for sex.

Masturbation is also associated with a host of health benefits, including lower stress levels, improved circulation to the pelvic region, and an increased likelihood of orgasm (alone and with a partner). It can help you to relax, promote mindfulness, and enjoy a good night's sleep—all of which will only serve to benefit your intimate relationship with a partner (e.g., fewer fights) and your sex life (more energy and confidence for sex). And of course, sleep is associated with many health benefits including improved cognitive functioning, digestion, healthy weight maintenance, and immunity.

SEDUCTION INSTRUCTION: SEXUAL SELF-LOVE

When was the last time you masturbated? And are you willing to give it a try today? We challenge you to put down this book (unless you find it erotic, in which case keep reading!) and think of something that turns you on. Reach down with your hands or toys and touch yourself. You don't have to orgasm to enjoy masturbation, but spend a few minutes touching yourself for pleasure to reap the rewards of sexual self-love—including being more open to being seduced.

In addition to practicing being touched and enjoying a solo sex session, you may also find that you need to practice being selfish. Everything we read and consume about sex tends to focus on performance. *Give a better blow job. Give them the hottest sex of their life. Give them multiple orgasms. What your partner really wants to hear in bed.* We've shifted from a culture of pleasure to a culture of performance. It's no wonder that most of us are not in the mood for sex.

If you really want to revolutionize your sex life and take care of yourself first, learn to be a taker. Ask for what you want—in and out of the bedroom. Get comfortable saying no and saying yes. Admit when you're not in the mood, and teach your partner what they can do to get you in the mood. It is okay to say, *I'm too tired, I'm going to sleep.* And it is okay to say, *I'm too tired, but if you kiss my neck and massage my lower back a little, I might get in the mood.* It is also okay to say, *I'm too tired, but I want you to go down on me.*

You might play the role of caregiver in every realm of your life, which can make it hard to accept offers and difficult to decline requests. But saying yes and no are essential sexual and relational skills that need to be cultivated both in and out of the bedroom, so we want you to practice right away.

SEDUCTION INSTRUCTION

▸ Identify one thing you normally say yes to but would prefer to decline. For example, do you have a neighbor who asks you to watch their cat and it is inconvenient, but you agree to do it anyway? Do your siblings ask you to host gatherings and cook at your house without reciprocating? Do you get pressured into volunteering beyond your capacity in your community or at school? Commit to saying no to at least one of these requests now. Send an email, pick up the phone, or write a text saying no. Once it becomes a habit, it will be freeing and will create more space for pleasure and fulfillment of all kinds.

▸ Identify one thing you normally say no to, but really wish you could say yes to. Does your partner offer you a massage after work, but you decline because do not want to put them out? Does your coworker offer you a ride to work, but you decline because you do not want to be a bother? Do you turn down offers of assistance at work because you want to do it on your own and play hero? Change this pattern now. Commit to saying yes to offers that appeal to you in your intimate relationship(s) and beyond.

> ▸ Say yes when you mean it and say no when
> you do not, without reservation. Hone this skill
> outside the bedroom first and you will get better
> at asking for what you want in the bedroom.

If you find that you're not in the mood when your lover tries to seduce you, ask yourself why. Perhaps you're tired or have other things on your mind. Be aware of your thoughts so that you can adjust them (if you want to get in the mood). Oftentimes, when we have a lot going on or when our sexual desire is not as high as our lover's, we shut sex and desire down entirely. However, you don't have to be immediately in the mood to push past these feelings and say yes to seduction. You can be receptive even if you're not in the mood (assuming you want to be). You can even challenge your partner to put you in the mood. If you shut the possibility of sex down before giving it a chance, you may miss out on potential pleasure and orgasm. Of course, you are not always required to say yes. But if you *want to* want sex, keep an open mind and allow seduction some time to lead to arousal and desire.

If you have difficulty shutting your brain off at the end of the day or you're distracted by work or kids, consider whether you are really prioritizing yourself and the relationship. Consider setting boundaries with coworkers and clients (e.g., turning on an email auto-reply after a specific hour), and acknowledge that your kids will be just fine if you invest in your relationship with your lover.

Couples who have been together for decades and still enjoy active, healthy sex lives tell us that it's essential to prioritize the relationship when the children are young. They say that while their friends prioritized their children, they put their relationship above their kids (much of the time). These couples realized that their kids would be all right and are, in fact, better off because they took time to invest in their coupled relationship. Even when their kids were young, they took nights off from cooking so that they felt rested (kids will survive if they eat takeout once in a while), and they escaped overnight for some adult time whenever possible.

How you allocate your time is up to you, but if you make excuses, you will continue to see the same results in your sexual relationships. If you want to shut down at the end of the night and connect with your partner, you will make the time to do so. We have clients who own and run businesses, take care of elderly parents, and raise multiple kids who also maintain happy relationships and hot sex lives, because they set time aside almost every day to invest in the relationships that matter most.

If you do not enjoy the way your partner(s) initiate sex, use positive reinforcement to highlight what you like and ask for what you want. For example, you might say, *I like how aggressive you are. I would really like it if you tickled my back first. You make me feel so loved when you put your hand right here like this.* Criticism will get you nowhere, so if your partner is making the effort to seduce you, show appreciation and give them credit for putting themselves out there, bearing in mind that you are not the one taking the initiative at this time.

SEDUCTION INSTRUCTION

The next time your lover attempts to seduce you, be honest about what you're feeling. Perhaps you push them away because you are angry about the fact that they don't help with chores; if this is the case, convey what you're feeling and *why* you're declining their advance. Perhaps you aren't in the mood because you're worried about a big presentation; ask them to give you a massage instead, and see where it leads (with no pressure to be sexual). Perhaps you find their approach off-putting; speak up and let them know how and when to seduce you.

Learning to be honest with regard to sex can be awkward, as you do not want to hurt your partner's feelings, and oftentimes, you don't fully consider *why* you're saying no. Reflect upon the last time you declined sex and jot down your reasons. Try to dig a little deeper and really think about what you were feeling—emotionally, physically, relationally, and generally. You do not need to overanalyze your sex life, but some consideration of why you do and do not desire sex will help you to better understand your own needs and convey them to your partner(s).

CONCLUSION

Before we sign off, we want to emphasize that sexual seduction and foreplay have no definitive start or end point. Together, we have covered a range of approaches, techniques, and strategies, but this is just the tip of the erotic iceberg. In experimenting with our suggestions, you have likely generated many more, and as technology advances, approaches to sexual seduction will continue to evolve. We look forward to learning and updating our tool kit alongside you, and we encourage you to keep exploring creatively and trying new things.

Seduction can be the pinnacle of pleasure, as it entails deep conversations, innovative ideas, vulnerable expressions, and expanding your comfort zone to be the best version of yourself. It is both an experience and a process. We are grateful that we have been a small part of this journey. Remember that the learning and growth will last a lifetime.

However you feel at this point in time, embrace it and know that we admire and appreciate you. We hope that you feel confident and competent in your ability to enjoy sexual seduction, foreplay, and all types of pleasure. We also offer a reminder that sexual confidence, pleasure, and fulfillment do not build linearly. You will experience fluctuations in the upcoming weeks, months, and years—this is perfectly normal, and it is a part of what makes sex so exhilarating and meaningful.

We are certain that you are equipped to master sexual seduction and foreplay *and* we recognize that mastery includes missteps, rejection, and even failure. Your willingness to embrace the celebrations alongside the challenges with an open mind makes you a better lover and a better person.

We wish you all the best in love, life, and sex.

Cheers to your sexual success!

FINAL SEDUCTION INSTRUCTION

Return to the questions you answered when you first picked up this book. Record your thoughts and answers in your journal today. Compare your answers and consider why some of them have changed over time. Consider returning to this activity again every few months, setting an alarm in your calendar as a reminder.

▸ How do you define sex?

▸ How do you think your lover(s) define(s) sex? Is this a conversation you have addressed or want to address in the future?

▸ How do you define seduction and foreplay?

▸ How do you think your lover(s) define(s) seduction and foreplay?

▸ What would you like to learn about seduction and foreplay?

▸ What do you find challenging about seduction and foreplay?

ENDNOTES

1   Sapolsky, Robert M. *Behave: The Biology of Humans at Our Best and Worst.* New York: Penguin Press, 2017.

2   University of Granada. "Study Confirms Importance of Sexual Fantasies in Experience of Sexual Desire." *ScienceDaily.* www.sciencedaily.com/releases/2007/06/070627223851.htm (accessed July 22, 2019).

    Birnbaum, G. E., Kanat-Maymon, Y., Mizrahi, M., Recanati, M., & Orr, R. (in press). "What fantasies can do to your relationship: The effects of sexual fantasies on couple interactions." *Personality and Social Psychology Bulletin.*

3   Leitenberg, Harold and K. E. Henning. "Sexual fantasy." *Psychological Bulletin* 117, no. 3 (1995): 469-96 .

4   Shoup-Knox ML, Pipitone RN. "Physiological changes in response to hearing female voices recorded at high fertility." *Physiol Behav.* 2015;139: 386–392. pmid:25449386

5   Hirsch, A; Gruss, J (1999). "Human Male Sexual Response to Olfactory Stimuli." *American Academy of Neurological and Orthopaedic Surgeons.* 19: 14–19.

6   Babin, Elizabeth Ann. "An examination of predictors of nonverbal and verbal communication of pleasure during sex and sexual satisfaction." (2013).

7   Chapman, B. P., Huang, A., Horner, E., Peters, K., Sempeles, E., Roberts, B. W., & Lapham, S. (2019). "High school personality traits and 48-year all-cause mortality risk: Results from a national sample of 26,845 baby boomers." *Journal of Epidemiology and Community Health*, 73(2), 106-110.

8   See generally: Curtis, Cate & Loomans, Cushla. (2014). "Friends, family, and their influence on body image dissatisfaction." *Women's Studies Journal.* 28. 39-56.

    L Michael, Shannon & Wentzel, Kathryn & N Elliott, Marc & Dittus, Patricia & Kanouse, David & Wallander, Jan & Pasch, Keryn & Franzini, Luisa & Taylor, Wendell & Qureshi, Tariq & Franklin, Frank & Schuster, Mark. (2013). "Parental and Peer Factors Associated with Body Image Discrepancy among Fifth-Grade Boys and Girls." *Journal of Youth and Adolescence.* 43.

    Webb, Haley J and Melanie J. Zimmer-Gembeck. "The Role of Friends and

Peers in Adolescent Body Dissatisfaction: A Review and Critique of 15 Years of Research." (2014).

9   See generally: Margana, Lacey, Manpal Singh Bhogal, James Edward Bartlett, and Daniel J. Farrelly. "The roles of altruism, heroism, and physical attractiveness in female mate choice." (2019).

Arnocky, Steven A., Tina Piché, Graham N. Albert, Danielle Ouellette, and Pat Barclay. "Altruism predicts mating success in humans." *British Journal of Psychology* 108 2 (2017): 416-435.

Farrelly, Daniel J., Paul Clemson, and Melissa Guthrie. "Are Women's Mate Preferences for Altruism Also Influenced by Physical Attractiveness?" (2016).

10   Ariely, Dan and George Loewenstein. "The heat of the moment: the effect of sexual arousal on sexual decision making." (2006).

11   Charmaine Borg, Peter J. de Jong. "Feelings of Disgust and Disgust-Induced Avoidance Weaken following Induced Sexual Arousal in Women." *PLoS ONE*, 2012; 7 (9)

12   Grewen, Karen M., Susan S. Girdler, Janet A. Amico, and Kathleen C. Light. "Effects of partner support on resting oxytocin, cortisol, norepinephrine, and blood pressure before and after warm partner contact." *Psychosomatic Medicine* 67 4 (2005): 531-8 .

Light K. C., Grewen, K. M. & Amico, J. A. (2005). "More frequent partner hugs and higher oxytocin levels are linked to lower blood pressure and heart rate in premenopausal women." *Biological Psychology*, 69(1), 5-21.

13   McDaniel, B. T., & Coyne, S. M. (2016). "'Technoference': The interference of technology in couple relationships and implications for women's personal and relational well-being." *Psychology of Popular Media Culture*, 5(1), 85-98.

14   Misra, Shalini, Lulu Cheng, Jamie Genevie, and Miao Yuan. "The iPhone Effect: The Quality of In-Person Social Interactions in the Presence of Mobile Devices." (2016).

15   Burleson, Mary H., Wenda R. Trevathan, and Michael J. Todd. "In the Mood for Love or Vice Versa? Exploring the Relations Among Sexual Activity, Physical Affection, Affect, and Stress in the Daily Lives of Mid-Aged Women." *Archives of Sexual Behavior* 36 (2007): 357-368.)

16   Dainton, Marianne, Laura Stafford, and Daniel J. Canary. "Maintenance strategies and physical affection as predictors of love, liking, and satisfaction in marriage." (1994).

17   Gulledge, Andrew K., Michelle H. Gulledge, and Robert F. Stahmannn. "Romantic Physical Affection Types and Relationship Satisfaction." (2003).

18   Anders, Sari M. van, Robin S. Edelstein, Ryan M. Wade and Chelsea R. Samples-Steele. "Descriptive Experiences and Sexual vs. Nurturant Aspects of Cuddling between Adult Romantic Partners." *Archives of Sexual Behavior* 42 (2013): 553-560.

19   Sonos. Music Makes It Home Study. Retrieved from https://music-makesithome.com/

20 Field, Tiffany Martini. "Touch for Socioemotional and Physical Well-Being: A Review." (2010). https://www.sciencedirect.com/science/article/pii/S0273229711000025

21 Turnbull, Oliver H., Victoria E. Lovett, Jackie Chaldecott, and Marilyn Doreen Lucas. "Reports of intimate touch: Erogenous zones and somatosensory cortical organization." *Cortex* 53 (2014): 146-154.

22 Leknes, Siri and I. Tracey. "A common neurobiology for pain and pleasure." *Nature Reviews Neuroscience* 9 (2008): 314-320

23 Turnbull, Oliver H., Victoria E. Lovett, Jackie Chaldecott, and Marilyn Doreen Lucas. "Reports of intimate touch: Erogenous zones and somatosensory cortical organization." *Cortex* 53 (2014): 146-154.

24 Holstege, Gert, Janniko R. Georgiadis, Anne Marinus Johannes Paans, L C Meiners, F van der Graaf, and Antje A. Reinders. "Brain activation during human male ejaculation." *The Journal of Neuroscience: the Official Journal of the Society for Neuroscience* 23, no. 27 (2003): 9185-93 .

25 Maxwell, Jessica A., Amy Muise, Geoff Macdonald, Lisa Catherine Day, Natalie O. Rosen, and Emily At Impett. "How implicit theories of sexuality shape sexual and relationship well-being." *Journal of Personality and Social Psychology* 112, no. 2 (2017): 238-279.

26 Herbenick, Debra L., Michael D. Reece, Devon Hensel, Stephanie A. Sanders, Kristen N. Jozkowski, and J. Dennis Fortenberry. "Association of lubricant use with women's sexual pleasure, sexual satisfaction, and genital symptoms: a prospective daily diary study." *The Journal of Sexual Medicine* 8, no. 1 (2011): 202-12.

27 Wimpissinger, Febu Florian, Karl Stifter, Wolfgang Grin, and Walter Stackl. "The female prostate revisited: perineal ultrasound and biochemical studies of female ejaculate." *The Journal of Sexual Medicine* 4, no. 5 (2007): 1388-93; discussion 1393.

28 Reece, Michael D., Debra L. Herbenick, Stephanie A. Sanders, Brian S. Dodge, Annahita Ghassemi, and J. Dennis Fortenberry. "Prevalence and characteristics of vibrator use by men in the United States." *The Journal of Sexual Medicine* 6, no. 7 (2009): 1867-74.

    Herbenick, Debra L., Michael D. Reece, Stephanie A. Sanders, Brian S. Dodge, Annahita Ghassemi, and J. Dennis Fortenberry. "Prevalence and characteristics of vibrator use by women in the United States: results from a nationally representative study." *The Journal of Sexual Medicine* 6, no. 7 (2009): 1857-66.